Make
Your Own
Skincare
Products

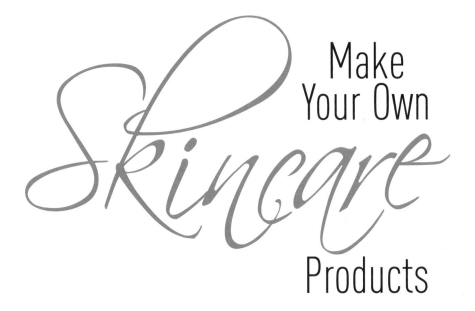

Make Your Own Skincare Products

SALLY HORNSEY

SPRING HILL

Published by Spring Hill, an imprint of How To Books Ltd
Spring Hill House, Spring Hill Road,
Begbroke, Oxford OX5 1RX
United Kingdom
Tel: (01865) 375794
Fax: (01865) 379162
info@howtobooks.co.uk
www.howtobooks.co.uk

First published 2011

How To Books greatly reduces the carbon footprint of its books
by sourcing all typesetting and printing in the UK.

British Library Cataloguing in Publication Data
A catalogue record of this book is available from the British Library.

ISBN: 978 1 905862 68 9

Produced for How To Books by Deer Park Productions, Tavistock, Devon
Designed and typeset by Mousemat Design Ltd
Edited by Jamie Ambrose
Printed and bound by in Great Britain by Bell & Bain Ltd, Glasgow

NOTE: The material contained in this book is set out in good faith for general guidance and no
liability can be accepted for loss or expense incurred as a result of relying in particular circumstances
on statements made in the book. Laws and regulations are complex and liable to change, and readers
should check the current position with relevant authorities before making personal arrangements.

Dedication

This book is dedicated to Ruby,
who is in search of perfect skin.

Contents

Acknowledgements

A big thank-you to everyone who supported me during the writing of this book. To my lovely team at Plush Folly, for keeping everything under control and always smiling when I walk into the office; to my friends and family, who unfailingly (or unwittingly!) tested the new product formulations; and to the Plush Folly bees, for providing the beeswax and honey used in the recipes.

Introduction

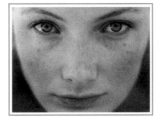

Recipes for skincare products can be found dating back many centuries – traditional recipes that evolved over time. Even in today's amazing world of advanced science, many of the original ingredients, such as clays, pumice, oils and herbs, are still used: such is their ability to make a difference to our skin.

Creating creams, lotions, toners, cleansers and other skincare products to suit your skin can be an exciting and challenging task. The rewards are enormous. Not only do you have the pleasure and enjoyment of designing and making the products, you also have the satisfaction and comfort of knowing exactly what ingredients you have used and how they benefit your skin. And benefit your skin they will – you'll be positively glowing!

The ingredients used throughout this book should be easy to find. Some are available from health-food shops and supermarkets; other, more specialist ingredients can be sourced online and I have included a list of suppliers of such ingredients at the end of the book.

Where possible, unprocessed, natural ingredients are used in the recipes. However, when I feel that a processed product – one that has been specifically developed to perform a function or target certain skin conditions – does a better job, I've included these, too.

Synthetic ingredients have to go through rigorous testing to ensure that they are skin-safe and have no likely adverse side effects, either short, or longer term. All finished skincare products, natural or otherwise, have to be assessed for safety by a qualified cosmetic chemist before they can be sold legally.

Weights & measures

Note that the ingredients used in making skincare products are often measured by weight, not by volume – including water. This makes it so much easier to be accurate. Essential oils are the exception here; because the quantities needed are so small, the oils are added drop by drop, otherwise the weight would be too light to register on most household scales.

Measuring chart

Use the following measurements as a guide in the event that your scales don't measure in small units. While the units shown below are not absolutely accurate, they do work as a guide and will enable you to make up the recipes in this book without rushing out and buying a new set of digital scales.

Quantity	Is roughly equal to
1ml	1g
5ml	1 teaspoon
10ml	1 dessertspoon
15ml	1 tablespoon
1ml / 1g essential oil	25–30 drops
30ml	1 fluid ounce
30g	1oz / ounce

Patch testing

Before using any of the finished skincare products you make, you should really consider carrying out a patch test. This isn't complicated, but simply involves placing a little of the product on the skin of the inner arm or on your neck, behind your ear.

If, after 24 hours, there is no redness, itchiness or adverse reaction to the product, then it is fine for you to use.

Shelf life of your homemade skincare products

Natural ingredients don't necessarily have the longevity and extended shelf life of synthetic products. If a finished product contains water, for example, its shelf life is considerably reduced and you should use it within a couple of weeks from the date you make it, unless you use a preservative. If your product does not contain water, then its shelf life will be much longer – usually at least 12 months from the date you make it.

The products made in this book all have a recommended shelf life listed as part of their recipe details, but this is very much dependent on the conditions in which you store your products and your ingredients. Please see the sections on storage, antioxidants and preservatives (pages 19, 25, 162 and 164) for more details.

Cosmetic regulations

The skincare products made in this book are for personal use only and must not be sold commercially. If you intend to make and sell cosmetic products, your product formulations must be tested and safety-assessed by a cosmetic chemist and conform to EU Cosmetic Regulations.

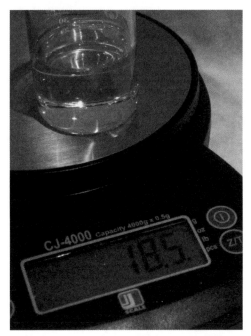

Accurate scales are a must when making your own skincare products

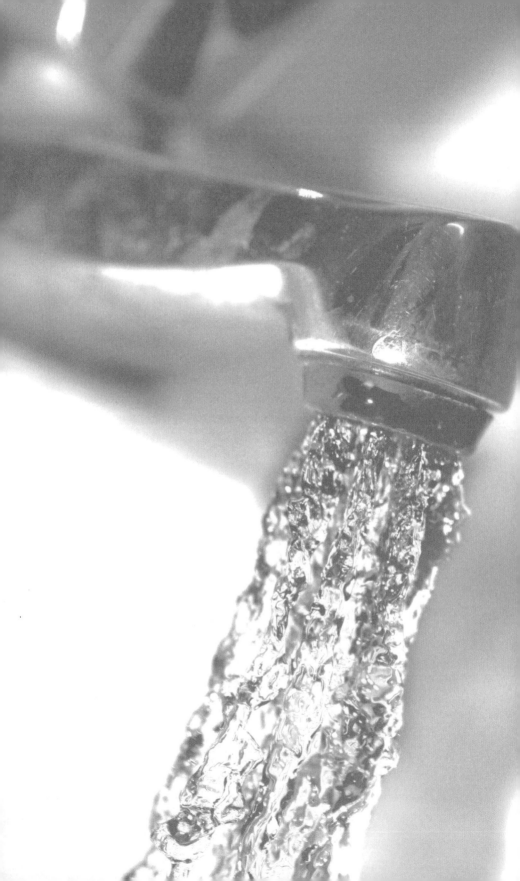

CHAPTER 1

Sensible Health & Safety

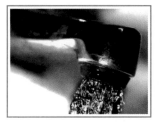

While it isn't compulsory to sterilise your equipment, you must ensure that your equipment, jars and bottles are clean, that your ingredients are stored in such a way that they will remain fresh and safe, and that you treat cleanliness as a priority.

It almost goes without saying that you should always wash your hands before embarking on any product-making activity. You may wish to wear protective gloves as well as an apron or other covering to protect your clothing.

Keep your equipment clean

Before using any utensil or equipment, make sure it is clean and dust-free. Wipe it round with a piece of kitchen paper or a clean cloth just to make sure. It isn't necessary to sterilise your equipment, but if you wish you can do so with the same sterilising solution and method used for sterilising a baby's bottle. Full instructions are given on the back of the sterilising solution containers available from most chemists.

If you don't wish to use sterilising solution, simply immerse your equipment into boiling water for 15 minutes, then leave to cool. Only do this, however, if you're certain that your equipment can withstand very hot temperatures.

Remember to clean any kitchen work surfaces with a suitable kitchen cleaner and antibacterial solution, both before and after creating your skincare products, to ensure the best-quality and longest-lasting results.

Handling cosmetic ingredients

Most of the ingredients used for making the recipes in this book are non-hazardous. However, they are oily and greasy and can make your hands and work surfaces slippery, so remember to clean up any spillage immediately and wash your hands when you've finished handling oily ingredients. Use an absorbent material, such as kitchen roll, to clean up spills, then wash over the area with a cloth soaked in hot, soapy water. Dry the area with a clean, dry cloth.

You will need a heat source, such as an electric hob, in order to warm up oils and waters as well as to melt butters and waxes. I recommend that you warm or melt all ingredients in heatproof jugs or bowls, which you then place in a pan of simmering water.

A Pyrex measuring jug (or similar) placed in a saucepan or baking tray of simmering water is easily the best (and most economical) method of melting and warming your ingredients. See Chapter 2, 'Tools of the Trade', page 22, for more information about heatproof equipment.

Safety precautions when using hot oils

When working with hot liquids or pastes of any sort, bear the following in mind:

- Heat oils, butters and waxes slowly. Heating them too quickly may allow them to get excessively hot and ignite.

- Never leave oils, or any other ingredients, unattended while you're warming or melting them; if oils get too hot they can catch fire. Hot oils can also cause severe burns if they come into contact with skin.

- Always turn saucepan handles inwards towards the centre of the hob. This prevents pans from being knocked off the stove or caught on a loose sleeve.

- Do not place flammable objects near the hob. Curtains, towels, cloths and food packaging can easily catch fire.

- Have fire-fighting equipment available in an easily reachable place. Fire extinguishers for all fire types and a fire blanket should be installed within reach of the cooker, but not so close that you couldn't get to them in the event of a fire.

• Make sure you have a fire alarm installed on the kitchen ceiling, or on a ceiling in the next room or hallway so that you, or anyone else in the house, can be alerted to any fire.

Safety precautions when handling essential oils

Essential oils are extracted from plants. They have a very intense, potent aroma and are too strong to be placed on the skin unless they have been diluted. They are widely used in many skincare products and are the basis of aromatherapy.

Obviously, you should keep all perfume ingredients away from children and pets. Essential oils have a wonderful scent, and some often smell like delicious food products. However, they are *not* edible, so never swallow or attempt to take the oils internally.

What is an essential oil?

Essential oils are plant oils that are volatile, meaning they are able to evaporate. Because they can evaporate, they are able to have an aroma – unlike other plant oils such as olive oil, sunflower oil and avocado oil. As essential oils evaporate, their molecules float into the air, around the room and up our noses.

Essential oil plant material

Many plants produce an essential oil, but some plants lack the ability to produce an aroma that can be captured in an oil. Essential oils can be extracted from different parts of a plant, such as the petals, leaves, wood, seeds, bark, roots and stems.

Essential oils not only bring an aroma to skincare products, but they also contribute active properties. An active ingredient is an ingredient that is considered to have an altering effect on the skin. Ingredients that perform a task such as self-tanning, exfoliating, moisturising, firming, rehydrating, etc., are all considered to be active ingredients.

Because essential oils are such potent little characters, they need to be treated and handled with extreme care, and the precautions outlined on the following page should be fully understood before starting your skincare product-making.

Essential oil safety checklist

Eye exposure
If any of the ingredients accidentally splash in your eye:

- Flush your eye with copious amounts of MILK for at least 15 minutes.

- Seek medical advice if painful stinging or reddening persists.

Handling
- Do not eat, drink or smoke when handling ingredients.

- Wash your hands before and after use.

- Avoid touching your face, especially your eyes and mouth, when you handle essential oils.

- Never apply the ingredients to inflamed or broken skin.

- Never use essential oils undiluted on skin.

- If you are pregnant, or have any underlying illness, seek medical advice before using essential oils.

Ingestion
If you do accidentally swallow any oils:

- Rinse your mouth with MILK, and seek medical attention immediately.

Spillage
- Clean any spillage with an absorbent material, such as kitchen roll.

- Remember to wear protective gloves, especially if the spill is excessive.

Storing cosmetic ingredients

- Store all cosmetic ingredients in a cool, dry place away from heat and direct sunlight.

- Store the ingredients in their original containers and make sure they are labelled so that the contents can be easily identified.

- Avoid contact with polished surfaces and plastic because the oils may damage or stain the surface.

- Keep an eye on the 'best before' or recommended shelf life of your ingredients and do not use them if they look odd or smell 'off'.

- Keep all the ingredients away from children and pets.

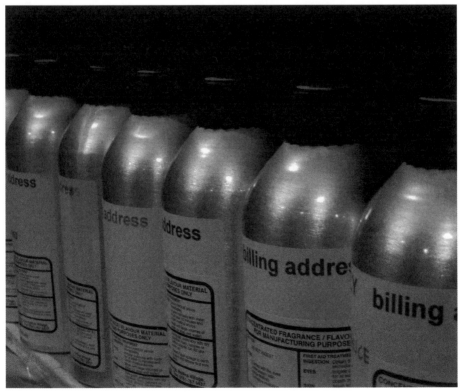

Essential oils can have an altering effect on the skin

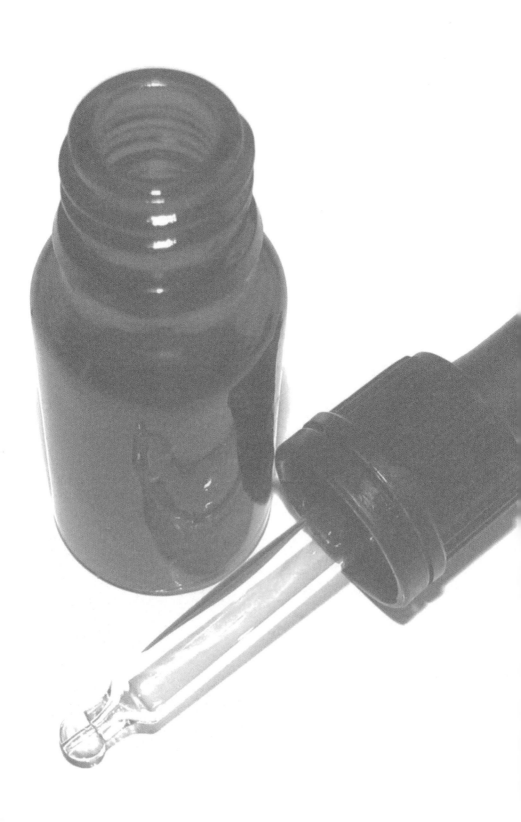

CHAPTER 2

Tools of the Trade

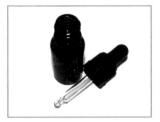

Making personal skincare products from home doesn't really require any specialist equipment. In fact, you may already have all the required equipment and utensils that are outlined in the following pages – so read through the lists, then check them against your store-cupboards!

However, regardless of whether you already own them or are buying brand-new items, I must emphasise the need to have everything thoroughly clean before use; *see* Chapter 1, 'Sensible Health & Safety', page 15, for advice. While this may seem as if I'm repeating myself, you cannot be too careful – especially where your health, and the health of your skin, is concerned.

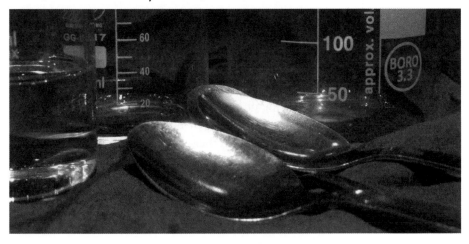

Heat proof beakers can withstand direct contact with heat

THE SKINCARE PRODUCT-MAKER'S TOOLBOX

Heat source

All hard oils, butters and waxes will need melting, and some ingredients will need warming up before use. Your standard hob can be used for this, but if you cook on gas, please make sure that you keep the heat down as low as possible.

Heatproof jugs & bowls

Stainless steel, glass or china heatproof bowls or jugs can all be used to heat and melt your ingredients. Pyrex glass jugs or bowls are perfect, because they can withstand direct contact with heat. We place our Pyrex jugs directly onto our hob (note that you can do this only on electric hobs, however; gas hobs are too unstable).

Pyrex jugs can be purchased at kitchen-utensil shops such as Argos, Sainsbury's and Tesco. If you can't find a source of Pyrex jugs, then any ovenproof bowl that can withstand heat will suffice, but these should never be placed directly on any type of heat source.

Saucepans & baking tins

If you're using bowls and jugs that can't be placed directly on a hob, then you can easily make yourself a double boiler – bain-marie style – with a saucepan or baking tin.

To make a double boiler, pour water in a saucepan or baking tray so that it comes approximately halfway up the heatproof bowl or jug; remove the bowl or jug. Heat the water to simmering and then turn the heat down as low as you can get it.

Put the ingredients in the heatproof jug or bowl and place the jug or bowl into the simmering water, being very careful not to let the water come into contact with the ingredients. Once the ingredients have warmed or melted, carefully remove the bowl or jug from the saucepan and take the saucepan off the heat. Do be careful because the jug or bowl may be very hot.

If you're worried about the heatproof jug or bowl sitting on the base of the saucepan and becoming too hot, turn another, smaller bowl upside down and place this in the larger saucepan. This will act as the base for your heatproof jug or bowl and prevent it from touching the base of the hot saucepan.

Bowls

You will need a selection of small bowls in which to mix your ingredients that don't require heating. Ramekins are ideal, and these can also go in the double boiler.

Scales

A set of digital scales are needed to weigh your ingredients accurately. Ideally these should measure in 0.5g increments and have a zero or 'tare' function (the latter allows the scale to account for the weight of the empty measuring container). If your scales don't go as low as 0.5g, then you can use the measuring chart on page 12 as a guide.

Spoons

You need a selection of spoons for dispensing and stirring. Stainless-steel teaspoons and dessertspoons are ideal.

A set of measuring spoons would be useful if you don't have a set of digital kitchen scales that can measure in small increments.

Spatulas

A spatula is very handy for getting the last traces of your creams and lotions out of the bowls. You will find using a small-headed spatula easier if your jugs and bowls are on the small side.

Protective clothing

To protect your clothing, always wear an apron and be aware that oil splashes can permanently mark cloth.

If you have long hair, you'll need something to tie it back with so that no stray hairs fall into your products.

Kitchen towel

Have a roll of kitchen paper handy to mop up any spills and splashes as soon as they occur.

PACKAGING YOUR SKINCARE PRODUCTS

The skincare products you make will need to be packaged in either a jar or a bottle, depending on the consistency and style of the product in question.

Jars and bottles can be glass or plastic, as long as they are clean and have tight-fitting lids. Make sure you store your empty containers with their lids on so that dust and fluff cannot fall into the jars or bottles.

Sourcing your containers

There are many beautiful perfume and cosmetic bottles and jars around, and if you enjoy trawling through junk shops and antique markets you may well find some beautiful secondhand containers to use. Old apothecary jars, especially those that are collectors' items, can be expensive, but with luck you'll find some that are beautiful without having a large price tag. Do check the jars over to make sure that the lid fits securely and that there are no obvious flaws in the sides.

No matter how old it is, it is imperative that you wash the container to remove all traces of product residue. To do this, wash the container in hot soapy water, then rinse it at least twice in clean hot water. Leave it to dry naturally. If you wish you can do a final rinse in a sterilising solution, such as Miltons. After sterilising, leave to drain and dry.

Sourcing what you want and in quantities that are manageable can often be a daunting task. If antique markets aren't your choice, then the internet is an excellent place to start your search for new bottles and containers.

When you find suppliers with reasonably priced, decently sized, perfectly shaped bottles and jars that are sold in individual units or small quantities, ask whether they will provide you with a sample if you plan to buy several bottles. If you're buying glass bottles, then a sample may not be necessary, but if you're buying plastic ones, then you should test the bottle to make sure it is suitable for your skincare products.

Please remember to label all your containers as soon as you use them. This not only helps identify the contents, but it also provides a date by which the product must be used.

STORING YOUR FINISHED PRODUCTS

As well as storing your cosmetic ingredients somewhere cool, dark and dry, your finished products will fare best if they are kept in these conditions, too. Most of us keep our skincare products on bathroom shelves or dressing tables, which means that our storage conditions aren't necessarily cool or dark.

If your container is opaque rather than transparent, then the product inside isn't exposed to direct light, which is good. If you keep your product in the fridge then it will be kept both cool and dark, but this isn't necessarily convenient.

As long as you store your products at no warmer than room temperature and use them regularly and within their shelf life, then they should be fine.

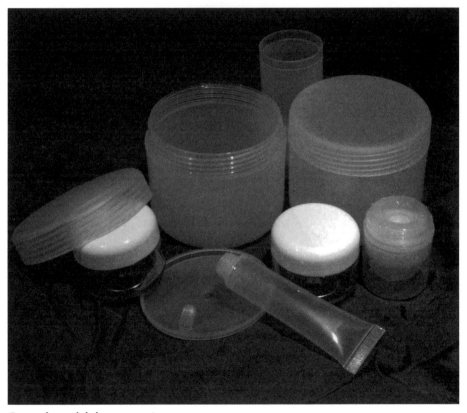

Remember to label your containers

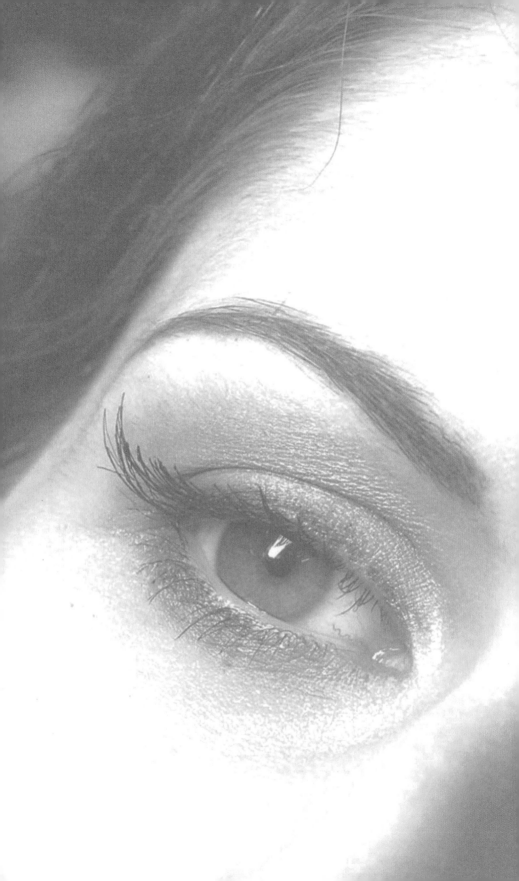

CHAPTER 3

Why Is Your Skin So Important?

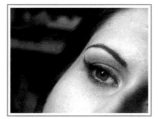

Your skin helps protect your body from dehydration and from injury and illness due to bumps, toxins, sunlight and viruses. It helps to control body temperature and acts as a sensor to inform the brain of changes to the environment, such as heat, cold, dry and wet. Skin keeps your muscles, blood and other bodily support systems in the right place – inside!

Your skin prevents vital body fluids from escaping at random. In addition, the role of managing the excretion of unwanted fluids and substances from the body is vital to your health. Since about 25% of all bodily waste exits the body via the skin, if your skin is not functioning properly, this will quickly become evident.

Skin: the largest organ

Skin is the body's largest, most versatile and extraordinary organ. It plays an important function that supports our survival. Skin can weigh up to 4.5kg and covers in excess of two square metres in most adults.

Without skin we wouldn't be able to feel. It is the body's largest sensory organ and allows us the sensation of touch.

Skin also has the most amazing shock-absorbing properties. It is waterproof, yet it can be washed over and over again while retaining most of its elastic quality. How amazing is that? Clothing manufacturers would love to be able to emulate this kind of functionality and resistance in fabrics!

THE STRUCTURE OF YOUR SKIN

As part of understanding how to treat your skin, you need an appreciation of how the skin is structured and how it works.

Skin is formed of three main layers: the epidermis, the dermis and the hypodermis. The epidermis is the outer layer of skin and this is subdivided into various layers.

Top skin layer – the epidermis

The epidermis is the surface of the skin and the bit that you can see. The thickness of the epidermis depends on your age and sex, but it is thicker in different areas of your body.

The sole of your foot, for example, is the thickest layer of all and is 30 times thicker than the skin on your eyelid. The average thickness of the skin on your eyelid is 0.05mm, while the average thickness of the skin on the soles of your feet is 1.5mm.

The epidermis itself contains several layers of skin. Starting with the deepest layer and working upwards to the outer layer, these are:

- the basal cell layer (*stratum germinativum*)

- the spinous cell layer (*stratum spinosum*)

- the granular cell layer (*stratum granulosum*), and

- the outer, clear/translucent layer (*stratum corneum*).

Basal cell layer

Your skin is in a constant state of self-renewal. The deepest or basal cell layer is one cell thick. These cells continuously divide, creating millions of healthy new skin cells each day. Some of these remain in the basal layer, dividing and creating new cells, while others migrate, passing up through the epidermis from the basal layer to the outer layer, pushing other cells upwards as they move.

The cells in the basal layer also produce melanin. Melanin is a pigment that gets absorbed by the dividing cells, giving them an element of protection against damage from ultraviolet light. The amount of melanin in your skin is dependent on your genetic background and also on how much your skin is exposed to the sun.

Spinous cell layer

The layer above the basal cell layer is called the spinous layer, also known as the 'prickle cell layer'. Cells passing through this layer change in shape from thin columns to polygons, and they start to produce keratin.

The main function of the keratinocyte cells is to form a barrier that helps protect the skin from infection, preventing unwanted matter such as bacteria, fungi or mould from penetrating it and entering the body. Keratin is a protein found in healthy skin, nails and hair.

Granular layer

The cells in the granular layer start to flatten out. It is here that waterproofing lipids are produced, along with more keratin.

Outer skin layer

Once cells reach the skin surface (*stratum corneum*), they flatten out, die and are gradually but continuously shed and replaced by younger cells pushed up from below. These older cells are strong and tough, ideal for holding us together!

The surface of your skin is only the thickness of a piece of paper, but it does a good job of protecting you and acting as a barrier to prevent water loss, among other functions. The outer layer of skin is exposed to ultraviolet light, which has an impact on the amount of melanin that is produced in the layers of your skin. Although you can block some ultraviolet light with suntanning lotions, your skin may still darken because the melanin brings about a change in pigment.

It takes roughly two weeks for cells to travel from the basal layer to the granular layer and a further 20–28 days to pass through into the stratum corneum. The entire process of replacing skin with new cell growth takes between four to six weeks, depending on your age, health and diet.

This period is a very important one to note. If it takes four weeks or so for your skin to renew itself, then any recently introduced skincare programme is also going to take that long before the full effect can take place. So… don't be disappointed if you don't see results from any skincare product straight away. You are working on promoting the growth of new, healthy cells, so you must allow four to six weeks for this to take place – and for you to notice the difference.

Middle skin layer – the dermis

The dermis lies beneath the epidermis and is connected by a continuous membrane. It is the thickest layer and is made up of collagen and fibrous, elastic tissue. It differs in thickness depending on the location of the skin on the body.

The dermis also contains nerve endings (these send messages to your brain and nervous system whenever you touch something), sweat and oil glands, hair follicles and blood vessels that carry oxygen and nutrients and take away waste.

The dermis is responsible for providing moisture to the epidermis. As well as moisture, the dermis produces other vital elements, all of which help to keep your skin in good working order. These are:

- collagen, to keep skin firm and strong,

- elastin, to keep skin flexible, and

- sebum, a natural oily secretion that keeps skin supple and moist.

Many skincare products include synthesised collagen and ingredients similar in structure to sebum to help boost that which is already produced by the dermis. The dermis gets thinner as we grow older.

Bottom skin layer – the hypodermis

The deepest and thickest layer of all is the hypodermis, also known as the subcutaneous layer. The hypodermis lies beneath the dermis and is composed of a huge network of connective tissue woven with fat cells.

The main function of the hypodermis is to store vital nutrients in the form of fat cells that provide insulation. While fat cells may not be the most popular part of your body, they do play an important role in insulating your body from changes in temperature, helping to keep your body temperature steady and constant. They also act as a shock absorber, helping to take the majority of impact from knocks and bumps.

The hypodermis is responsible for giving skin its curves and general shape, as well as cushioning and protecting the outer layer. It also connects the skin to essential tissues and muscles, feeding and draining the blood vessels which connect it to the outer layers of the skin.

The hair on your skin starts life in the subcutaneous layer, making its way up and through the dermis, the epidermis and out into the air, poking out from your skin. These hair follicles rely on the skin's natural oil, sebum, to make the hair flexible, waterproof and shiny, and as the hair travels through the dermis, it coats itself with a layer of nourishing sebum.

THE FUNCTION OF SKINCARE PRODUCTS

In a nutshell, the function of skincare products is to feed, protect and repair your skin. If you achieve all three functions as part of your skincare routine, then you'll be rewarded with healthy, glowing, fresh-looking skin.

Like tending to plants in a garden, looking after your skin is an ongoing process. Your skin requires different management and treatments at different times of the year, and at different stages of your life. Each item in a skincare portfolio has a different role. From cleaning to plumping, hydrating to smoothing, every product in this book has been chosen specifically to perform a part in your overall beauty-management strategy.

Treatments for skin

This book includes everyday and specialist skincare treatments that are easy to make and, if used regularly and as directed, will make a difference to your skin, both in the short- and longer term.

Cleansers

Cleansing not only removes dirt, bacteria, make-up, excess sebum and dead skin cells, but it also unclogs pores and helps the skin to breath.

Toners

Toners are used to remove the remains of any cleanser, oil, dirt and other debris from your skin. A toner is an astringent and will therefore also help to cool and refresh your face, close open pores and restore the skin's pH acidity levels.

Moisturisers

Moisturisers have one of the most important roles to play in skincare. Their aim is to strengthen and mimic the body's own naturally produced sebum and protect the skin against moisture loss. A good moisturiser will rehydrate the skin, making it feel supple and soft with improved elasticity, without making it feel greasy or look shiny. A moisturiser also creates a barrier, helping to protect skin against dirt, grime and pollution in the air. Moisturisers can penetrate the surface layer of skin and to deliver therapeutic active ingredients to it.

Specialist treatments

Specialist treatments are designed to target particular problem or needy areas. Treatments include gels, which are cooling, refreshing and soothing balms, which are ultra-hydrating and will help to alleviate itching and quench patches of dry skin, and serums, which help to increase suppleness and soften the skin.

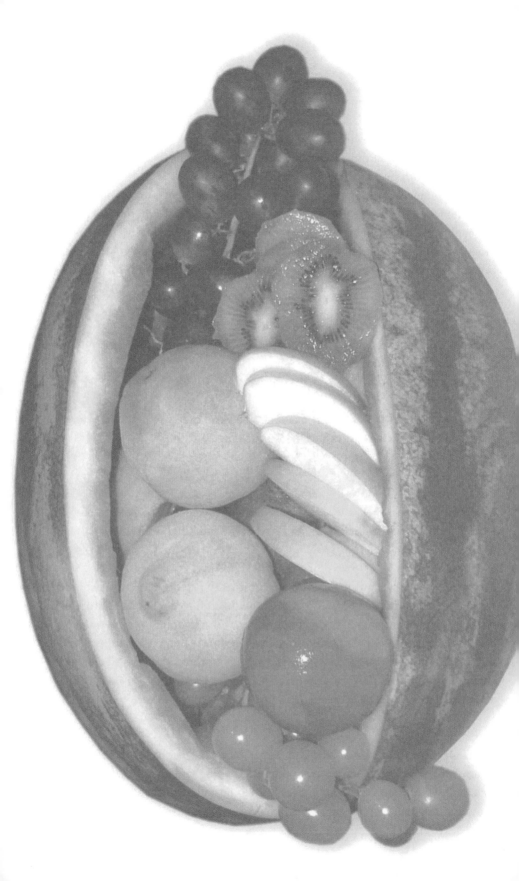

CHAPTER 4

Caring for Your Skin

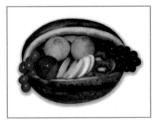

With such an amazing protective covering to our body, we should do what we can to nurture and care for our skin.

To achieve a healthy, glowing skin you need a combination of three things: a healthy diet, plenty of exercise and a good skincare programme. While this book doesn't include details about a healthy diet and a regular exercise plan, it does contain all you need to know about designing and making bespoke skincare products and choosing the best cosmetic ingredients to help keep your skin healthy, glowing and beautiful.

In order to create appropriate skincare products, first you need to be able to identify your particular skin type. Changes in the environment – such as temperature and humidity – together with changes to your body brought on by hormones, fitness levels, age and lifestyle, can all have an impact on your skin, and its health and appearance. By determining what skin type you have, you can then formulate products that will best support it when coping with all these external factors. This chapter shows you how to do just that.

DIFFERENT SKIN TYPES

'What is my skin type?'

This is one of the hardest questions to answer. Most of us have the tendency to believe that we have sensitive or combination skin, or oily skin in the summer and dry in the winter – but in fact our skin type is totally reliant on the amount of natural sebum our body produces.

Normal skin

The appearance of healthy, normal skin is that of having a smooth, even skin tone that is free from imperfections or shiny or dry patches. It has a matte finish and a soft, silky feel.

Strangely enough, though, normal skin isn't 'the norm'; it is rarely seen on anyone other than young children – and a few, very lucky, adults.

Oily skin

The appearance of oily skin is generally shiny, with large, open pores. Oily skin also tends to have a slightly thicker texture than normal skin, due to an increased activity of the sebaceous glands. Oily skin is prone to spots, blemishes, pimples and blackheads because the open pores can become congested with a build-up of dirt and grime.

Oily skin is caused by overactive sebaceous glands producing more oil than is necessary to protect the skin. On the plus side of things, oily skin tends to age slower than other skin types due to the higher levels of sebum that keep it lubricated and hydrated.

In addition to genetic factors, oily skin can be triggered by an overzealous or harsh cleansing routine.

Combination skin

The appearance of a combination skin type is an oily area across the forehead and down the nose and chin which is known as the 'T-zone' due to its T shape. The skin in the T-zone is typical of oily skin and is prone to enlarged pores and pimples. The areas on the cheek, however, are susceptible to dry patches.

Sensitive skin

The appearance of sensitive skin is a thin, fine texture that tends to redden easily. It reacts quickly even to slight changes in temperature. Sensitive skin is prone to patchy redness and rashes with dry, flaky areas.

Sensitive skin is very delicate and more inclined to allergic reactions. It will also burn in the sun and wind very easily. Sensitive skin reacts to beauty products containing certain dyes, fragrances, chemicals and other irritants. Other triggers can be changes in weather, temperature, stress and pollution.

Dry skin

Dry skin is usually rather pale-looking and lacking in shine. It is likely to have pinker patches accompanied by occasional dry, flaky, scaly areas which indicate a lack of moisture. It can feel rough and dry to the touch and often feels itchy and tight.

Since this skin is so dry and therefore delicate, it is the first to show wrinkles around the eyes and mouth area. Dry skin can be caused by lack of hydration to the skin, possibly through diet as well as lack of moisturising creams or the wrong type of skincare routine.

DETERMINING YOUR SKIN TYPE

If you're unsure what type of skin you have, there is a very simple test you can do to analyse your skin type called the skin-blot test.

The skin-blot test

This very simple procedure effectively measures the amount of oil on your skin.

At the time of the test, remove all traces of makeup from your face and gently rinse with tepid water. Pat your face dry with a clean towel and sit calmly and quietly for ten minutes.

Take four small pieces of tissue paper such as acid-free tissue paper, lens-cleaning tissue paper or facial blotting paper, and press one piece onto your nose, another piece onto your forehead, another onto your chin and the final piece onto a cheek. Do not rub; just press against the skin gently and hold for eight to ten seconds.

Carefully let go of the piece of paper. If a piece of paper sticks to an area of your face when you let go, or comes away with an oil mark on it, you have skin prone to oiliness.

However, if the oily area was part of your T-zone (forehead, nose and chin), then check the piece on your cheek as well. If this has no oily mark on it, then it is likely that you have a combination skin type.

If the pieces of tissue come away without any problem and have no marking on them then you have a dry skin.

Just to throw confusion into the pot, normal skin types may or may not pick up an oily patch on the tissue. I believe you'll know if you are a normal skin type because you will have little trouble with your skin, seldom break out in pimples or dry patches, hardly ever have oily patches or blackheads and constantly maintain a natural dewy complexion. Lucky you!

This skin-blot test will determine what type of skin you have at any particular moment. Do bear in mind though, that there are factors that may temporarily change your skin type.

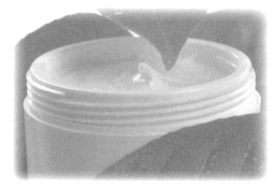

CONDITIONS THAT AFFECT YOUR SKIN

While your skin type and sebum production are likely to be hereditary, a number of conditions can affect your skin temporarily, either in the short or longer term. Recognising how your skin changes during the seasons, at busier, more stressful times, and during natural cycles of your body, will assist you in understanding what skin treatments will help alleviate any adverse skin complaints.

Hormone levels

It is likely that your skin will become oilier and prone to pimples during your period, whereas skin tends to become drier during menopause. Hormone changes throughout pregnancy can also bring about a change in sebum production.

Weather conditions

The sun and heat can make skin oilier because they cause the sebaceous glands to create more sebum. During the winter, or in windy weather, your skin can dry out and become flaky. Just think, for example, of how chapped your lips get in the winter.

Diet

What you eat and put on the inside will ultimately have an impact on how you look on the outside.

Exercise

Give your skin a healthy glow by getting your blood pumping around your body to increase oxygen flow and drain away toxins. If you can't find the time or inclination to go to the gym, a brisk walk three times a week for 20 minutes does wonders.

Medication

Certain medicines can temporarily change your skin type, especially hormone-balancing medications.

Stress

Being stressed can have an impact on your immune system, making your skin more vulnerable to infections, and possibly eczema. Being stressed may also cause you to have a broken sleep pattern, which results in puffy skin, especially around the eye area.

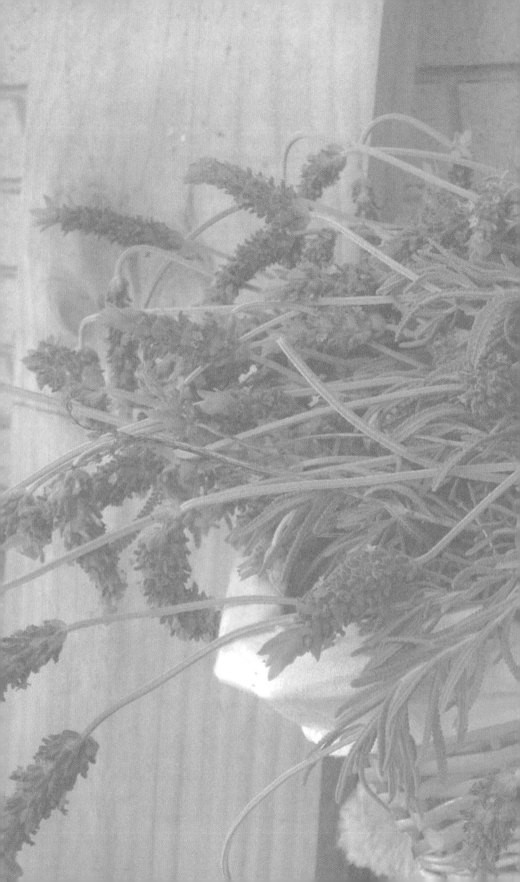

CHAPTER 5

Cosmetic Ingredients

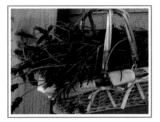

The individual ingredients used in making cosmetic products are selected to bring specialist functionality, beneficial properties and superior skin-feel. Understanding what each ingredient does, how it performs and how it interacts with others will enable you safely to design and create your own skincare products.

Skincare products contain a range of ingredients, including waxes, butters, oils, powders, waters, fragrances and herbs. These bring with them a wealth of vitamins, essential fatty acids and minerals, as well as antibacterial, anti-inflammatory, hydrating and other beneficial qualities to smooth, soften, calm, moisturise, plump, clean and generally treat your skin.

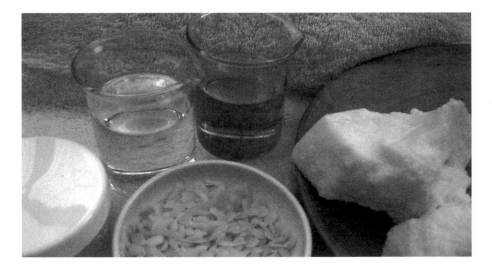

ACTIVE INGREDIENTS

An active ingredient is an ingredient that is considered to have a dermatological effect: that is, an altering effect on the skin. Ingredients that perform a task such as self-tanning, exfoliating, moisturising, firming, rehydrating, etc., are considered to be active ingredients. Common types of active ingredients include essential fatty acids, vitamins, enzymes and alpha hydroxy acids (AHAs).

The term 'active ingredients' is a contemporary buzz phrase, and many products are advertised as having active ingredients. In fact, most skincare products contain active ingredients and always have. For example, a popular active ingredient in eye gel is witch hazel – which for decades has been known to soothe and cool skin.

The effectiveness of any ingredient depends on whether it penetrates your skin sufficiently, which in turn depends on whether there is enough active ingredient in a product and whether you're applying it properly. Massaging your moisturising product into your face, for example, always helps it to penetrate further.

Warm skin absorbs ingredients better than cold skin, and because a large number of active ingredients penetrate better when dissolved, consider splashing warm water on your face and patting it with a warm towel to dry off some of the water before applying a moisturiser. This will leave your face warm and damp – the perfect canvas on which an active ingredient can thrive.

The quantity of your active ingredient should be 10%+ in order to have an effect. This doesn't mean that stuffing your skincare product full of an active ingredient will make it work better. The quantity included should work with the other ingredients to feel comfortable and safe on your skin.

Many active ingredients have a short shelf life and can become ineffective or even harmful if stored too long and exposed to the air. The beauty of hand-made personal skincare preparations is that you can make them in small batches to be used straight away, therefore minimising the time they're exposed to the air.

Essential fatty acids
Essential fatty acids are found in vegetable oils such as olive, evening primrose and avocado oil. Essential fatty acids fall into two categories:

- Alpha linolenic acid (LNA) (omega-3) and
- Gamma linoleic acid (GLA) (omega-6).

These essential fatty acids are required to maintain a good level energy, circulate the blood, produce haemoglobin, help keep a healthy, balanced sebum production and prevent skin from becoming dry.

Alpha linolenic acid – omega-3
Our bodies are unable to produce or store essential fatty acids so it is vital that we absorb them regularly via some form. A good approach is both to ingest them and to apply them topically. Oils rich in omega-3 include kukui, flaxseed, safflower, sunflower, soybean, peanut and walnut oils.

Gamma linoleic acid – omega-6
Gamma linoleic acid (GLA) is an omega-6 unsaturated fatty acid. The main sources of GLA are evening primrose, borage, hemp and flaxseed oils. GLA helps reduce water loss from the epidermal layer and therefore reduces the chances of eczema and psoriasis, which it can also help to soothe. Oils rich in omega-6 include argan, kukui, flaxseed, soybean, sunflower, sesame, safflower and rapeseed oils

Vitamins in skincare
Vitamins in food products are known for the benefits they bring in terms of health and a properly functioning body. They are just as important in skincare products.

Vitamin C
Scientific research shows that vitamins C and E can penetrate the top epidermal layer and are absorbed into the skin. The degree of penetration depends on their concentration and how they are applied. Vitamin C has antioxidant properties which help protect the skin from sun damage, and it can help stimulate the cells in the dermis to produce collagen.

Vitamin A
Vitamin A, also known as retinol, is required for healthy growth and repair of skin tissue and so it helps maintain a healthy skin. It encourages and stimulates the growth of collagen, which keeps skin firmer. Vitamin A improves the ability of the skin to resist itches and irritation as well as protecting it against sunburn. Retinoic acid is derived from vitamin A and it helps minimise wrinkles, smooth rough skin and fade age spots.

Vitamin A is found mainly in food, but high traces are present in carrot seed essential oil, rosehip oil and pumpkin seed oil, all of which can be used in moisturising creams and preparations.

Vitamin E
Like vitamins A and C, vitamin E (tocopherol) is an antioxidant and is often used with other oils to prevent them from becoming rancid. It is found in base oils such as wheatgerm and avocado oils. Vitamin E is both natural (d-alpha tocopherol) and synthetic (dl-alpha tocopherol), and the natural oil is twice as effective as its

synthetic partner. Vitamin E helps improve skin healing and can reduce age spots, and it is an ideal ingredient to use in skincare products for maturing skin types.

Vitamin D

Vitamin D helps keep skin healthy and is a powerful antioxidant. Coconut oil, hemp oil, flaxseed oil and sunlight are natural sources of vitamin D.

Enzymes in skincare

Enzymes are found in raw vegetables, nuts, seeds and fruit. Skincare products containing these raw ingredients will benefit not only from the presence of enzymes but also from their antioxidant, vitamin and mineral contents.

Enzymes help speed skin renewal, improve and smooth skin texture, reverse sun damage and can be used to treat acne. Fruit is a rich source of enzymes. Look for dried fruit, fruit extracts and fruit oils such as strawberry oil, which can be included in skincare products.

Alpha hydroxy & other acids

Alpha hydroxy acids (AHAs, sometimes referred to as fruit acids) are believed to be beneficial to the skin. Alpha hydroxy acids can help to reduce skin wrinkling, improve elasticity and skin texture by reversing some of the aging processes as they slowly exfoliate the top layer of skin, revealing the fresher, healthier-looking skin underneath. More importantly, alpha hydroxy acids encourage and stimulate the growth of new skin cells. There are various types of alpha hydroxy acids. These include:

• *Glycolic acid* The most common type used in skincare. It comes from sugar cane and is used in chemical peels and serums because it has strong exfoliation properties.

• *Lactic acid* has deep hydrating properties and is a popular ingredient in commercial moisturising creams. Lactic acid can be found in dairy products and can be used in handmade cosmetics very easily by using the dairy powders, such as buttermilk powder or yoghurt powder, in face masks.

• *Salicylic acid* Technically speaking, salicylic acid is not actually an alpha hydroxy acid, even through it is usually grouped with glycolic and lactic acid. Salicylic acid comes from fruits and plants such as willow bark and is considered a beta hydroxy acid because it works deeper into the skin to unblock pores and reduce lines.

USING ESSENTIAL OILS

Many common ingredients can be used to bring an abundance of active properties to handmade skincare products. The simplest of these include essential oils, base oils and butters.

Essential oils are active ingredients, meaning they will bring about a change to your skin by improving its appearance or helping to clear up a skin problem. There are oils that are astringent, such as lemon essential oil, that will help treat oily skin, and oils that are hydrating, such as rose essential oil, which will help treat dry skin. There are oils that help promote cell regeneration (frankincense) and therefore help mature skin, and oils that help to heal (lavender) and can help treat burns, spots and infections.

If you use two essential oils that have opposite capabilities – for example, rose and lemon – rather than clear up a dry or oily skin, they will cancel each other out, but if you enjoy the aroma of lemon and rose, then you will still benefit from the uplifting fragrance of the oils. Some essential oils, such as ylang-ylang, are suitable for both oily and dry skin because they help regulate the production of sebum.

Essential oil suitability for different skin types

Use this chart to help you decide which essential oils, or blend of essential oils, you should include in your skincare products. There are far more essential oils available than those shown in the list, but this reflects those I feel bring particularly good skincare benefits to your products.

Dry	Oily	Combination	Spotty	Mature	Sensitive
Rose	Lemon	Geranium	Petitgrain	Frankincense	Rose
Chamomile	Lime	Ylang-ylang	Grapefruit	Neroli	Chamomile
Neroli	Petitgrain	Lavender	Juniper Berry	Rose	Lavender
Sweet Orange	Lemon Grass	Neroli	Lavender	Myrrh	Patchouli
Patchouli	Juniper Berry	Rosewood	Patchouli	Sandalwood	Sandalwood
Sandalwood			Myrrh	Ylang-ylang	Rosewood
Ylang-ylang			Tea Tree	Rosewood	

Properties of essential oils used in skincare

While the list on the previous page is useful for making a quick decision on which essential oil(s) to use, the chart shown here gives you a little more information as to how the oils can help with particular skin conditions.

Essential Oil	Benefits of oil when used in skincare products
Bergamot	•Treats minor wounds and cuts and can soothe rashes
Oily Skin	•Uplifting, antidepressant, refreshing
Carrot Seed	•Rejuvenating effect; smoothes and softens
All skin types	•Stimulating, warming
Cedar	•Relieves itchiness and helps balance oily skin
Oily skin	•Aphrodisiac, soothing, antidepressant
Chamomile	•Very soothing for dry skin and irritating rashes
Dry and sensitive	•Soothing, calming
Clary Sage	•Balances and adjusts the production of sebum
All skin types	•Aphrodisiac, relaxant
Eucalyptus	•Healing, clears congested skin, anti-inflammatory
Oily skin	•Refreshing, stimulating; aids concentration
Frankincense	•Reduces oil production, rejuvenates skin, encourages new skin-cell growth;
All skin types,	soothing, healing
especially mature	•Soothing; meditation aid
Geranium	•Soothes burns and sore patches, reduces bruising, improves blood circulation
Normal and	and helps balance over-/underproduction of sebum
combination skin	•Uplifting, balancing, soothing
Grapefruit	•Helps with lymphatic drainage to remove toxins. Unclogs congested skin
Oily skin	•Uplifting, anti-stress, antidepressant
Juniper Berry	•Anti-inflammatory; unclogs congested pores
Oily skin	•Calming; encourages positive thoughts
Lavender	•Treats wounds, burns and sore patches. Soothes itchy skin
All skin types	•Soothing, calming, uplifting
Lemon	•Clears congested pores, astringent, antiseptic
Oily skin	•Refreshing, uplifting, antidepressant

Essential Oil	Benefits of oil when used in skincare products
Myrrh *All skin types*	• Healing, soothing, hydrating, anti-infection • Calming; focuses the mind
Neroli *Combination and* *mature skin*	• Helps improve skin elasticity; stimulates cell renewal and regenerates skin • Aphrodisiac, uplifting, antidepressant
Orange (Sweet) *Dry, normal, oily* *and mature skin*	• Helps with lymphatic drainage to remove toxins. Soothes dry skin, promotes collagen formation to help skin become firmer • Cheering, uplifting, warming
Petitgrain *Problem skin*	• Decongests blocked pores, healing • Relaxing , soothing, calming, antidepressant
Patchouli *All skin types*	• Renews and regenerates skin cells and tissue. Fights general and fungal infections. A great all-purpose skincare ingredient • Aphrodisiac, warming, relaxing, sensual
Rose *Dry, mature* *and sensitive skin*	• Rehydrating, reduces redness and inflammation • Aphrodisiac, antidepressant, uplifting, soothing
Rosewood *All skin types,* *especially sensitive*	• Rejuvenating, targets wrinkles, soothing • Soothing, uplifting, steadying
Sandalwood *All skin types*	• Rehydrating, superb for dry and chapped skin and balancing oily skin • Soothing, antidepressant, sensual
Tea Tree *Problem and* *oily skin*	• Known for its antiseptic qualities. Useful for treating spots, pimples and infections • Warming, uplifting
Ylang-ylang *All skin types*	• Balances the secretion of sebum • Aphrodisiac, antidepressant

Essential oil quantities

Essential oils are extremely potent and can often be irritating to the skin. Used in sensible and small quantities, however, they will enable your products to work on various ailments and skin disorders while bringing a wonderful aroma that won't be overpowering.

When making your own skincare products it is important to know how much essential oil can be used safely in any recipe. The maximum limit I suggest is 0.5% for facial products, but you may find that even at this level, the aroma is rather strong for a product you'll be wearing on your face.

Skincare products fall into two camps: those that are left on and those that are rinsed off. For example, a cleanser and a face mask are rinse-off products, whereas moisturising creams, balms and serums are leave-on products. Rinse-off products can be formulated with more than 0.5% if you wish, but I would always err on the side of caution initially and stick with a lower level.

Calculating the amount of essential oil to use

A little maths for you now! In order to work out what 0.5% of your product is in terms of weight or volume, you need to know the total weight or volume of your product.

Let's say that your moisturising cream is made up of water, wax and oils and that the total weight of the water, wax and oils is 200g. This total weight – 200g – is the value of 100%. You can now work out the value of 0.5% by using the following calculation:

In this example, the total weight is 200g and you want to calculate 0.5%. Therefore the calculation is:

$$200 \div 100 \times 0.5 = 1$$

The calculation tells you that 0.5% is equal to 1g, therefore you should use a maximum of 1g essential oil in your product.

Calculating smaller quantities

If you're making only a small pot of a product, your total weight may be much lower than 200g. For example, if you're making a face mask and want to make enough for only one treatment, the recipe will be something along the lines of 15g clay, 15g water, 2g oil.

Let's perform that calculation again, but this time on the smaller total face-mask weight. The total weight of the face-mask ingredients is 32g. Using the calculation above, the maths would work out like this:

$$32 \div 100 \times 0.5 = 0.16$$

So this time you can see that you need to use 0.16g of essential oil in your face mask. Now, unless you have scales that can measure tiny increments, measuring 0.16g will be difficult. However, using the measuring chart shown earlier on on page 12, you can work out how many drops of essential oil there are in 0.16g.

The measuring chart tells you there are approximately 25–30 drops of essential oil in 1g. Using that equation, you can calculate how many drops equal 0.16g. To do this, divide 0.16 into 30. The answer is 4.8, so you need 4.8 drops, which you can round down to 4 drops (always err on the side of caution).

Your face mask recipe made using 15g clay, 15g water and 2g oil will require a maximum of 4 drops of essential oil if calculating your essential oils at 0.5%.

Storage & shelf life of essential oils

As with all cosmetic ingredients, store your essential oils somewhere cool – and preferably dark. While essential oil containers are often labelled with a 'best before' date, you don't necessarily have to stick to that date; very often the oils are still fine to use beyond it.

Provided you've stored them properly, some oils are fine after many years. In fact, some, such as patchouli and vetiver, actually improve with age. Citrus oils have the shortest shelf life, but even these can be used beyond their usual 12-month recommendation.

A simply way to check on the viability of an essential oil is to smell the bottle. If the oil still smells fresh, then it is probably perfectly OK.

USING FLORAL WATERS

A floral water is a by-product of essential oil processing. It is the water that is collected when plants are distilled to extract oils. Floral waters are also known as flower waters, hydrolats, distillates and hydrosols.

During the steam-distillation process, steam absorbs much of the aroma and beneficial qualities of the plant itself. As the steam cools, it condenses into water, with small quantities of essential oil dispersed within it. Once the essential oil has been extracted, the remaining water is bottled and forms delicately perfumed floral water.

Some steam distillation uses the same water for several distillation cycles. This makes the floral water stronger in both aroma and therapeutic property than one created from a single distillation. As therapeutic materials, floral waters bring beneficial properties to skincare products. Many recipes in this book call for spring water, but you can use a floral water instead without changing the quantity of water required.

Floral water uses

Apart from the lovely, refreshing, cooling feeling you get from splashing or spritzing a floral water onto your skin, you will benefit from the same therapeutic qualities found in the essential oil that was extracted from it.

Some floral waters smell bitter or earthy and not necessarily like the plant they've been extracted from, or their essential oil equivalent. The therapeutic qualities are the same, however; because the water is diluted, it's safe to use directly on skin. Floral waters are an excellent alternative to essential oils and can be used in many different ways.

Natural toners

Floral waters make fabulous toners. Take advantage of the therapeutic qualities and use floral waters, or a blend of floral waters, for your particular skin type and condition.

Spritz

Put a floral water into a spray bottle and refresh yourself with a cooling mist. Remember to keep your eyes shut when spraying your face, though!

Aftershave

Certain floral waters can be used to soothe shaving rash and calm the skin. Lavender is perfect for this and will leave a mild scent on the skin.

Hair rinse

Rosemary water keeps hair healthy and shiny. Use as a final rinse after shampooing and conditioning.

Mouthwash

Gargling with peppermint water freshens breath, while gargling with tea tree water is good for soothing sore throats.

Laundry

Freshen your laundry with a spray of your favourite floral water. You can also use floral waters in the iron.

Insect repellent

Eucalyptus and geranium floral waters make great insect repellents.

Decongestant

Spray eucalyptus and peppermint waters onto your pyjamas or handkerchief or directly onto your chest to help you breath easily at night when you have the snuffles.

Refresh tired eyes

Place a little rose or lavender floral water onto cotton-wool pads and place over your closed eyes for 15 minutes or so.

Floral water suitability for different skin types

Use this chart to help you decide which floral waters, or blend of floral waters, you should include in your skincare product. As stated before, whenever a recipe calls for spring water, you can use any of the waters below instead. Alternatively, make up a solution that is part spring water and part floral water and use this in your recipe.

Dry	Oily	Combination	Spotty	Mature	Sensitive
Rose	Petitgrain	Geranium	Petitgrain	Frankincense	Rose
Chamomile	Lemon Grass	Ylang-ylang	Juniper Berry	Neroli	Chamomile
Neroli	Juniper Berry	Lavender	Lavender	Rose	Lavender
Ylang-ylang	Lemon	Neroli	Tea Tree	Ylang-ylang	Sandalwood

Storage & shelf life of floral waters

Store floral waters in a cool, dry area, avoiding contact with bright sunlight. If stored in this way, they should have a shelf life of 18 months or so. Any spoilage of the waters will be from air and heat. It is perfectly acceptable, although not absolutely necessary, to keep opened bottles of floral waters in the fridge. See the chapter on making infusions, page 133, for details on how to make your own version of plant waters to be used in cosmetics.

USING BASE OILS

Oils are the foundation ingredients in handmade skincare products. Oils such as olive, avocado and sunflower are known as base oils, carrier oils, fixed oils or vegetable oils. These oils have been extracted from part of the plant but they differ from essential oils in that they have no noticeable aroma and are safe to go on skin without diluting them beforehand.

Base oils are sometimes referred to as carrier oils because they carry essential oils (or other ingredients) on the skin, diluting them so that they are at safe levels for skincare products. Carrier oils play a key role in diluting essential oils, which are otherwise too strong to put directly on skin. Essential oils disperse in base (carrier) oils and can then be massaged onto the body. I shall refer to these oils as base oils so as not to confuse them with essential oils.

Base oils are obtained from seeds, nuts, fruits, vegetables and leaves and are used as a base to which other ingredients are added. Olive oil, for example, is extracted by cold-pressing olives. The result is a beautiful greeny-gold oil, and while it may have a hint of olive about it, it is known for its emollient and culinary qualities rather than its aroma. Strawberry seed oil is similar, in that it is obtained by cold-pressing the seeds. This yields a beautiful golden oil that is similar in texture to olive oil. Strawberry seed oil will not smell of strawberries.

Base oils can be used on their own without the addition of other ingredients and can be applied to the skin as a massage oil or as a moisturiser. They can also be blended with all other base oils.

Most base oils are in liquid form, but occasionally they're solid – coconut oil is one example of a solid base oil. Solid oils have a high volume of stearic fatty acid, but it's possible to remove this to render the oil more liquid. This is why coconut oil comes in both solid and liquid forms; the latter should be referred to as 'fractionated coconut oil'.

Understanding the different properties and characteristics of these base oils is very important, because these will become the building blocks of your skincare products. If you think that using sunflower oil will bring the same benefits as using avocado oil, or that wheatgerm oil will give you the same feel as if you had used rice bran oil, then think again! Base oils feel and behave differently, and this will have an impact on your final skincare products.

Behaviour & characteristics of base oils

Base oils are composed of triglycerides and fatty acids and typically contain monoglycerides and diglycerides. It is these fatty acids, such as alpha linolenic acid and linoleic acid, that make up the characteristic of the oils and give them different qualities and skincare benefits.

Just as importantly, it is the feel of the oils and the way they behave on your skin that makes some better than others for use in skincare products. Oils are typically thought of as being thick and greasy, but for many this is not the case at all.

Long oils

There are occasions where you want to spend time applying a skincare product without it being absorbed quickly into the skin. An example of this is a cleanser: you want to spend time massaging it on your face while it picks up dirt and grime.

Grape-seed oil is a useful base oil for such occasions. It is absorbed fairly well into the skin, but not too quickly. This also makes it an ideal choice for a massage, since there is plenty of 'rubbing' time without having to stop and apply more oil.

Short oils

Short oils, also known as on-and-gone oils, are oils that absorb into the skin very quickly and thoroughly, leaving no greasy residue. Take a little avocado oil and rub it into your arm. After a very short time the oil has vanished, because it has been fully absorbed into your skin, leaving no greasy residue.

Avocado oil has total absorption ability, and on top of that, it is *quick* to be absorbed. This makes it a superb oil to include in skincare products where you want to apply a cream that is quickly absorbed by the skin without having to rub too much. A facial moisturiser is a prime example of this, where a little massaging is acceptable, but quick absorption is a necessity.

When designing your skincare products, you need to understand how each oil works in terms of speed and thoroughness of absorption, but also what properties it will bring to a product.

Base oil characteristics

Use the chart below as a guide to which oils to use in your products. For example, if you're formulating a face cream for someone who has dry skin, consider including evening primrose and jojoba oil in your formulation. Both these oils are fully absorbed into the skin.

Evening primrose is absorbed quickly, whereas the jojoba oil is absorbed at a medium speed, which means it will take a little extra time to massage it into the face, otherwise it may be a bit shiny for a while. The list covers a range of different base oils but is by no means definitive.

Base oil	Especially suitable for	Particular qualities and benefits in skincare products	Absorption		Shelf life
			Speed	Ability	
Almond (Sweet)	All skin types	Nourishing, rejuvenating, soothing oil. Anti-wrinkle, anti-inflammatory.	Medium	Medium	2-3 years
Apricot Kernel	Sensitive, dry, mature	Nourishing, anti-inflammatory, soothing and especially good for sensitive and mature skins.	Medium	Medium	2-3 years
Argan	Dry, mature	Immensely hydrating, protective and helps keep skin supple. Rich source of vitamin E.	Quick	Total	3 years
Avocado	Dry, mature	Anti-wrinkle, encourages skin cell regeneration, healing. Rich in vitamins A, B_1, B_2, B_5, D and E.	Quick	Total	3 years
Blackcurrant Seed	All skin types	Anti-inflammatory, boosts immune system. Healing, protecting. A rich source of omega-6 and fruit enzymes.	Quick	Total	2 years
Castor	Dry, mature, oily, problem	Provides protective barrier, soothing, cleansing, antifungal, anti-inflammatory and healing.	Slow	Hardly any	2 years

| Base oil | Especially suitable for | Particular qualities and benefits in skincare products | Absorption | | Shelf life |
			Speed	Ability	
Coconut	Dry, mature	Protects, softens, soothes, anti-inflammatory. Rich source of vitamin D.	Slow	Medium	5 years
Evening Primrose	Dry, mature	Anti-wrinkle, encourages skin-cell regeneration, soothing. Treats dry, chapped skin. Rich in omega-6.	Quick	Total	6-12 months
Flaxseed	Dry, mature, problem	Rich source of omega-3 and vitamins D and E. Anti-irritant and anti-inflammatory. Helps dry, chapped skin, scarring, age spots.	Medium	Medium	6-12 months
Grapeseed	All skin types, oily	Refines pores, firms, nourishes. Rich source of omega-6, vitamin E. Helps mature, damaged, tired, stressed skin.	Slow	Good	1 year
Hazelnut	Dry, oily	Astringent, good for oily skin, toning, rebalancing, soothing.	Medium	Total	3 years
Hemp Seed	Mature, problem	Rich source of omega-6 and vitamin E. Soothing, restorative, anti-inflammatory, healing.	Quick	Total	6-12 months
Jojoba	Combination, dry, oily, problem	Helps treat acne. Soothes sensitive skin. Suitable for all skin types. Antioxidant, conditioning, rich in vitamins and minerals.	Medium	Total	5 years

Base oil	Especially suitable for	Particular qualities and benefits in skincare products	Absorption		Shelf life
			Speed	Ability	
Kukui Nut	Dry, mature	Protecting, rejuvenating and conditioning. Rich source of vitamins A, C and E. Suitable for very dry, chapped skin, acne and sore areas.	Quick	Total	1 year
Macadamia Nut	Dry, oily, mature	Anti-wrinkle, hydrating, soothing, protective, healing and anti-irritant.	Medium	Total	3 years
Melon Seed	All skin types	Healing and protecting. Rich source of vitamin C, omega 3 and 6.	Quick	Total	2 years
Olive Oil	Dry, mature, sensitive	Anti-inflammatory, anti-wrinkle, heals, conditions, firms, softens. Rich in proteins, minerals, vitamins.	Medium	Medium	3 years
Peach Kernel	Dry, sensitive, mature	Anti-wrinkle, anti-inflammatory, rejuvenating and regenerative. Rich source of vitamins A and E.	Medium	Medium	2-3 years
Rapeseed	All skin types	Rich source of omega-6 and vitamin E.	Medium	Medium	6-12 months
Rice Bran	Dry, sensitive, mature	Nourishing, conditioning, anti-inflammatory, antioxidant, anti-wrinkle and skin-softening. Rich source of vitamin E.	Medium	Total	2-3 years
Rosehip	Problem, dry, mature, sensitive	Healing, hydrating, anti-wrinkle and useful at reducing scarring. Rejuvenating, regenerating and a rich source of vitamins A and C.	Quick	Total	6-12 months

| Base oil | Especially suitable for | Particular qualities and benefits in skincare products | Absorption | | Shelf life |
			Speed	Ability	
Safflower	Mature, sensitive, dry	Soothing, moisturising, anti-inflammatory. Rich source of omega-3.	Medium	Total	1 year
Sunflower	All skin types	Nourishing, conditioning, skin-softening and pore-refining. Rich source of vitamins A, D and E, omega-3 and 6.	Medium	Medium	2 years
Vitamin E	All skin types	Antioxidant, will help to minimise damage caused by sun and environment such as skin pigmentation marks, fine lines and wrinkles. Very hydrating.	Slow	Medium	5 years
Walnut	Dry, mature, oily	Soothing, hydrating, regenerative, toning, firming and anti-wrinkle. Rich source of vitamins A, C and E.	Quick	Total	2 years
Wheatgerm	Mature, dry	Soothing, hydrating, anti-aging and regenerative. Suitable for very dry, flaky skin. Rich source of proteins, vitamins A, D and E.	Medium	Medium	2 years

Storage & shelf life of base oils

Bottles of oils don't often come with a 'best before' date on the label, but oils need to be stored correctly in order to give them the maximum shelf life possible. If suppliers were to state a 'BBE' (Best Before End) date and you found the oils were past their best at an earlier date due to not being stored correctly, this could kick off a dispute between you and the supplier.

Oils only have a good shelf life if stored properly in cool, dark conditions without too much exposure to air. Always keep the lid on the bottle when not in use and keep the oils in a cupboard away from a heat source.

A rancid oil will smell musty and crystallise around the neck of the bottle. If an oil has gone rancid, it is no longer suitable for use and needs to be thrown away.

Extending the shelf life of your oils

Adding up to 10% vitamin E to your oils will prolong their shelf life since vitamin E is an antioxidant and helps slow the oxidation process that makes them go rancid.

Add 10ml vitamin E to a 1-litre bottle of your shorter shelf-life base oil and give it a good shake. Don't forget to mark the label on bottle so that you know it now contains vitamin E (tocopherol) as well as the original base oil.

Adding vitamin E in this way will give your short-shelf-life oils an extended shelf life of between 18 months to two years. The oil will still need to be stored somewhere cool and dark, of course.

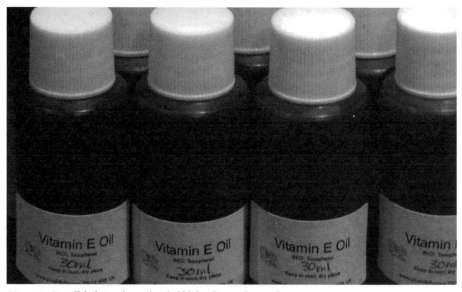

Vitamin E will help prolong the shelf life of some base oils

USING BUTTERS

Butters are used in conjunction with or instead of oils. They have the same ability to moisturise and have a range of active properties, each useful for skincare products. Unlike oils, they are solid and have an impact on the final texture and thickness of your product.

Butters can be applied directly to the skin, but because they are very rich and intense, it is often felt they're too heavy and need to be mixed with other ingredients to make them more skin-friendly in terms of texture. All the butters listed below are suitable for treating dry, cracked and chapped skin.

Many varieties of butters are used in cosmetics; many of them are exotic and not that easy to source. While I love the hydration capabilities of butters such as illipe, kokum, murmuru, tacuma and cupuacu, the butters I've selected for the chart below are also lovely to use – and easier to get hold of.

Butter	Particular qualities and benefits in skincare products	Absorption		Shelf Life
		Speed	Ability	
Cocoa	Very hydrating and skin-softening. Protective, antioxidant and anti-wrinkle. This butter is extremely hard and has a high melting point. Rich source of vitamin E. Extracted from the cocoa bean, it gives off a slight hint of chocolate.	Slow	Medium	5 years
Mango	Moisturising, anti-wrinkle, anti-itch and improves skin elasticity. A rich source of vitamins A and E. Semi-solid at room temperature but melts on contact with skin.	Slow	Medium	2 years
Olive	Antioxidant, anti-inflammatory, conditioning, firming, hydrating and nourishing.	Slow	Medium	2 years
Shea	Protective, hydrating, skin-softening and soothing. A rich source of vitamins A and E. Shea butter would be one of my chosen ingredients if I were stranded on a desert island...	Medium	Medium	2-3 years

Storage & shelf life of butters

Although they are semi-solid at room temperature, it is advisable to store butters in a lidded container, and if you have space in the fridge then fill it with your butters. Suppliers often dispatch butters in polythene bags, which may suffice if the transportation is in a chilled van, but on a hot day I've taken delivery of a bag of liquid oil!

Stored somewhere cool and away from direct sunlight and strong odours, your butters should have a shelf life of at least two years, longer for cocoa butter.

USING WAXES

Waxes are used in cosmetics to thicken, harden and emulsify creams and salves and to moisturise, protect and soothe the skin. Waxes are too hard to be applied directly to skin and will need melting before they can be mixed with other cosmetic ingredients.

A number of different natural waxes are available, and apart from an emulsifying wax, they all have a similar function in skincare products. Beeswax is my preferred choice because it has so many wonderful properties that help soften, moisturise and generally treat the skin. I have selected three different waxes, listed below, for use in the recipes in this book.

Wax	Particular qualities and benefits in skincare products	Absorption		Shelf life
		Speed	Ability	
Beeswax	Nourishing, antibacterial, relieves itching. Soothing and hydrating.	n/a	n/a	5 years
Jojoba wax	Processed from jojoba oil and therefore offering the same properties as the oil: antioxidant, conditioning and rich in vitamins and minerals.	n/a	n/a	5 years
Emulsifying wax	Processed from vegetable oils, often coconut. A vital ingredient in creams and lotions made from waters and oils.	n/a	n/a	5 years

Emulsifying wax

There are many variations of emulsifying waxes available, and while they all bind and hold water and oils, they may also bring other properties to a product in terms of skin feel, hydration ability and cream-thickening capability. They are usually used at a rate of 4–18%, depending on the thickness you're trying to achieve for your final product.

While some emulsifying waxes may produce a very thick cream at 10%, others may require at least 15% before a cream will stand up in peaks. If in doubt, ask your supplier for advice – or simply have fun experimenting.

The emulsifying wax used in the recipes in this book is emulsifying wax NF (National Formulary), which is used extensively and is widely available.

Storage & shelf life of waxes

Store waxes in a lidded container away from heat and strong aromas. Waxes are pretty robust and have a long shelf life.

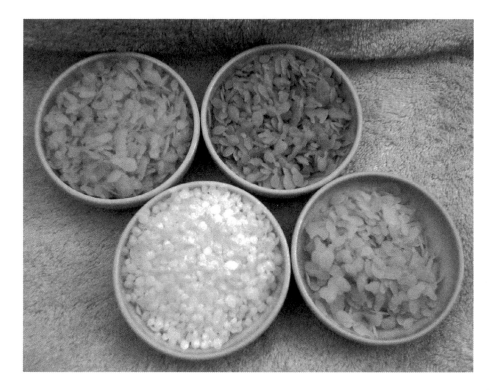

SPECIALIST INGREDIENTS

Some of the recipes in this book call for slightly more unusual or specialist ingredients. The following have been chosen to treat a particular skin condition, for their wonderful therapeutic properties or simply because they make the skincare product work better. The supplier list at the end of the book on page 172 will help you source these ingredients.

Ingredient	Particular qualities and benefits in skincare products	Products	Shelf life
Aloe Vera *Function: healing, cooling, refreshing liquid or gel*	Nature's first-aid plant, aloe vera is cooling, healing and refreshing. In its liquid form, it can be used as part-replacement for any spring water or on its own. In gel form, it can be used to replace a xanthan gum gel.	Cleansers, creams, face masks	18 months –2 years
Bamboo Powder *Function: exfoliating ingredient*	A natural exfoliating powder, rich in mineral salts and silica, which can help strengthen skin tissue. bamboo powder gives a gentle scrub, so it makes an ideal exfoliating ingredient.	Scrubby cleanser	2 years
Clays and Muds *Function: deep cleanse, detox, provider of nutrients*	Clays and muds are interchangeable. Their function is to draw out impurities and excess oils from the surface and just below the surface of the skin. Clays and muds are dried in the sun and are a valuable source of concentrated minerals such as oxides, magnesium, calcium, potassium, dolomite, silica, manganese, phosphorous, silicon and copper, all of which help to construct a strong, healthy skin. Dead Sea mud also improves circulation, deep cleanses and detoxifies, softens and relieves itchiness.	Face mask	2 years
Emulsifiers *Function: binds and holds water and oils*	Emulsifiers are needed to bind and hold oils and waters. Without an emulsifier, these two ingredients will separate. For creams and cleansers I use an emulsifying wax (emulsifying wax NF) and for liquid products containing water and oils, sucragel or polysorbate.	Cleansers, creams and lotions	2 years

Ingredient	Particular qualities and benefits in skincare products	Products	Shelf life
Fruit and Dairy Powders *Function: provides enzymes, alpha hydroxy acids, lactic acid, vitamins and other nourishing elements*	Spray dried-powder form of fruits can be used in face masks. These have all the benefits of the original fruit and are rich in vitamins and amino acids. Dairy powders include dried milk, dried buttermilk and dried yoghurt. While the fresh versions of the fruits and the dairy products can be used, the shelf life is reduced to a few days.	Face masks	1 year
Glycerine *Function: moisturiser, good skin feel*	Glycerine is a humectant (a substance that helps a product retain water) and will give an extra hydrating boost because it attracts moisture from the air and locks it onto the skin's surface. Glycerine also gives 'glide' to your scrub, allowing it to slide across your skin without tugging. Cleansers, moisturisers, toners.	Cleansers, moisturisers, toners	2 years
Ground Nut Shells *Function: exfoliating ingredient*	Crushed nut shells are one of the original exfoliating ingredients. Shells such as almond shells, apricot kernel shells and ground walnut shells give an interesting speckled texture to your scrubs, but they can be a little coarse.	Scrubby cleanser	
Honey *Function: Skin softener, moisturiser*	Honey is a humectant, meaning that it will grab moisture from the air and lock it onto skin. Honey will help soften and moisturise your skin. Often difficult to include in facial skincare products, so honey powder is a suitable alternative.	Face masks, cleansers	2 years
Jojoba beads *Function: Exfoliating ingredient*	An alternative to bamboo powder, jojoba beads are tiny jojoba wax esters coated in a way that leaves them with rounded sides – and therefore no sharp edges.	Scrubby cleanser	2 years

Ingredient	Particular qualities and benefits in skincare products	Products	Shelf life
Mica/Glitter *Function:* *visual appeal* *via colour* *and sparkle*	Mica is a skin-safe, shimmering powder that comes in many different colours. While it forms the basis of mineral make-up products, it is also used to colour creams and gels. Cosmetic-grade glitter can add a sparkle to any product.	Creams, gels	5 years
Olive Squalane *Function:* *luxury* *moisturiser*	A very hydrating natural liquid derived from olives. Silky and light, this easily penetrating, anti-aging liquid can be used directly on the skin, blended with oils, and included as a key ingredient in luxury creams.	Creams, serums, gels	5 years
Preservatives *Function:* *extends shelf* *life of products*	Used to prevent the growth of bacteria, mould, fungus and yeast in products that contain water.	Aqueous creams, lotions	2 years
Seaweed: Kelp and Spirulina *Function:* *adds nutrients,* *colourant*	Seaweed is rich in minerals, making it a useful addition to any scrub or face mask. Powdered kelp can be used with sea salt to give your scrub a 'marine' theme. Spirulina is a lovely green-turquoise colour and is a natural colourant for many cosmetics.	Face masks, scrubby cleansers	12 months
Sugar *Function:* *exfoliating* *ingredient*	Soft dark/light brown is the softest of the sugars and is suitable for use as a gentle scrub.	Scrubby cleansers	2 years

Ingredient	Particular qualities and benefits in skincare products	Products	Shelf life
Tinctures *Function: provides various active properties depending on botanical infused*	Made by extracting the properties from herbs and flowers into oils and water (infusion) and alcohol (tinctures).	Cleanser, creams, toners, masks	A few weeks/ months
Xanthan gum *Function: thickener, moisturiser*	A gelling ingredient used to make a gel or give added thickness or viscosity to products.	Face masks, gels, creams, toners	5 years
Zinc oxide *Function: soother, healer*	A white powder used to soothe and heal rashes. Provides protection from the sun and has an SPF of 5 upwards, depending on the percentage used in creams. Difficult to use as a higher factor, however, because the powder also acts as a whitener and in larger doses will work like white face paint!	Creams, balms	5 years

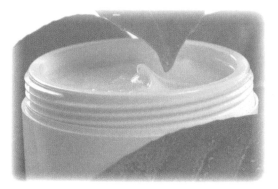

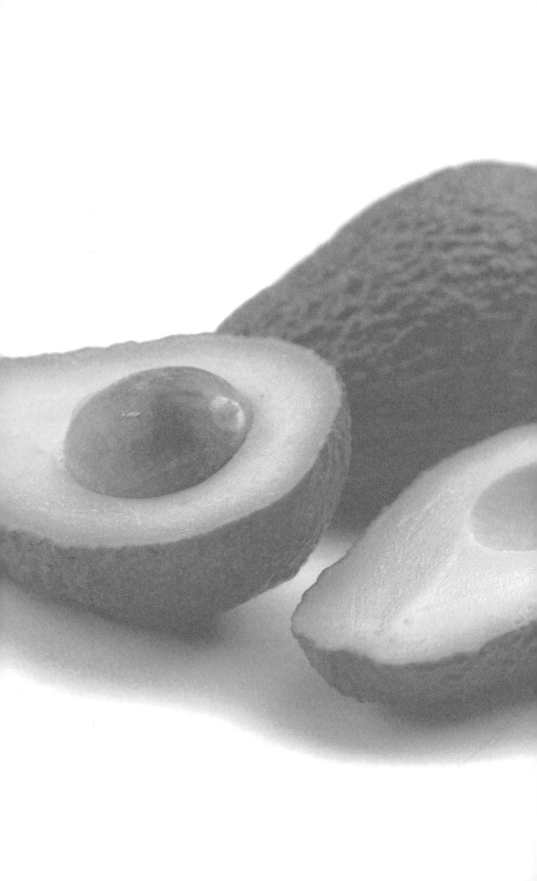

CHAPTER 6

Making Facial Products: Routines & Recipes

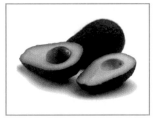

As mentioned previously, to achieve a healthy, glowing complexion you need a combination of three things: a healthy diet, plenty of exercise – and of course a good skincare programme.

The best skincare programme means taking some basic steps on a regular basis that are easy for you to maintain and suited to your lifestyle. Ideally your skincare routine should consist of a daily and a weekly programme, although you should be careful not to overdo it and disturb the skin's normal function any more than is necessary.

Your skin is self-cleansing and self-nourishing from the inside; your skincare routine should be designed simply to give it a helping hand.

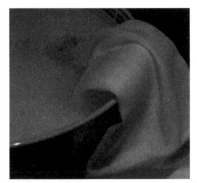

Cleansing will help to dislodge and remove traces of dirt, makeup, bacteria and excess oil from your skin

CLEANSING

You need to cleanse your skin in order to remove dirt, grime and excess oil accumulated during the day. Cleansing is vital. It not only removes dirt, bacteria, make-up, excess sebum and dead skin cells, but it also unclogs pores and helps your skin to breathe. It doesn't matter how tired you are, you should never go to bed without first cleaning your face – not only because traces of make-up will transfer to your pillow, but also because the make-up and dirt left on your skin may clog your pores, causing sebum build-up and the possibility of spots. Your poor skin! It's trying to rest and renew while you're sleeping, and yet you'll be making it work very hard if you force it to deal with stale make-up and dirt.

Cleansing should be a gentle yet thorough process. If you wear a lot of make-up, then cleansing may take longer, because you need to remove the make-up first before you cleanse your skin.

Types of cleansers

Cleansers come in the form of either a creamy cleanser or liquid oil cleansers, both designed to be massaged onto the face and then wiped off with cotton wool, a tissue or muslin. A good cleanser will pick up all traces of make-up and grime from your skin, which is then removed when the cleanser is wiped off. A creamy cleanser is usually suitable for all skin types. This type of cleanser can also be placed onto a piece of cotton wool or tissue and wiped across the face, collecting dirt and make-up.

Foaming cleansers consist of a gentle liquid soap which is rubbed onto the face with a little water. This produces a foam that helps to break down make-up and grime, which is then removed when the cleanser is rinsed away.

How & when to cleanse

Ideally you should cleanse your face twice daily: once before you go to bed and once again in the morning to prepare your face for the day. Cleansing your face should take approximately two to three minutes.

To cleanse, tie your hair back away from your face. Take a little of the cleanser on your clean fingers and place a little blob on your chin, each cheek, forehead and tip of your nose. Using the tips of your fingers, lightly massage the creamy cleanser onto all areas of your face. Massage the skin gently – you're doing this to increase the blood and oxygen circulation.

Remember that time and gravity pulls everything downwards, so you should help defy gravity by using gentle sweeping movements that go across and up your face from chin to forehead. This will help keep your skin's tissue firm and uplifted.

If you're applying the cleanser to your face with a cotton-wool pad or tissue, rub it in small, circular movements, making sure you cover every inch of your face. Avoid the delicate eye area if the cleanser isn't suitable for eyes. If your cleansing lotion is gentle enough for eyes, sweep a pad across each eye from inner corner to the side of your face. Clean your eyelashes with a downwards then upwards movement, being very careful not to get any of the cleanser in your eye.

If you have a problem area on your face, use a separate cotton-wool pad to clean it. Don't risk contaminating other areas of your face by using the same pad all over.

Wipe off residue cleanser with a tissue or cotton-wool pad and rinse with water. Pat dry using a soft, clean towel.

Hot-cloth cleansers

Use a hot muslin cloth to wipe cleanser off your face. Run the muslin under hand-hot water, squeeze out any excess water and use it to remove the traces of cleanser from your face.

You can use the cloth as a gentle exfoliating treatment at the same time by rubbing it in little circular movements on different areas of your face – this is especially useful for getting into the crevices around the side of your nose. Rinse the muslin cloth after use.

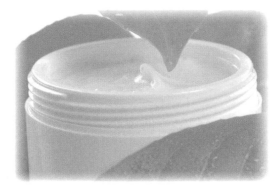

Cleanser recipes

In this section, I've included a selection of cleanser recipes ranging from creamy to exfoliating cleansers. At the end of each recipe is a list of suggestions on how to vary the recipe to make it suitable for different skin types while still using the same method to make your cleansing product.

If you're used to washing with a soap cleanser, then you may be surprised not to find a foamy cleanser in the recipe section. Foaming agents, such as sodium lauryl sulphate, sodium laureth sulphate and disodium cocoamphoacetate (look for them on the ingredients listing on your foaming cleanser product) are included in commercial products to ensure that the products froth and create a foam. These are often a little drying for your skin – which is precisely why I haven't included them.

If you prefer a lathering cleanser, your best bet is to use a natural handmade soap that has olive oil and shea butters as its base ingredients. This will give you a natural foamy wash without drying out your skin.

Oil cleansers

Oil cleansers may seem a little out of the ordinary if this isn't your usual method of cleansing. Sadly, today we tend to wash our face with harsher cleansers which rid our faces of oil as well as make-up, grime and general dirt. Our skin then has to work hard to replenish the oils needed to keep it lubricated, supple and healthy; often it overcompensates by producing too much oil.

By using an oil cleanser, you're still able to remove unwanted make-up and dirt, but you help your skin by not stripping it completely of precious oils. Your skin will still be clean, and after a few weeks of using this style of cleanser, it will look healthier and positively glowing.

Sucragel is a light emulsifier derived from sugar and oils, and its function in the cleanser recipes is to make it easier to remove traces of cleanser when toning or rinsing.

TOTAL WIPEOUT BALANCING CLEANSER

For combination skin

The total wipeout cleanser is excellent for combination skin, with its jojoba and geranium essential oils. Jojoba oil is very similar in structure to the skin's own sebum, and therefore, on oilier areas, tricks the sebaceous glands into thinking that they are overproducing sebum and so need to slow down. On drier areas jojoba oil helps to bring much-needed moisture. Geranium essential oil helps to regulate sebum production. Geranium can often be a little sharp and spicy in aroma, so if you prefer a softer aroma, try rose geranium as a suitable alternative.

60g jojoba oil
30g sunflower oil
8g sucragel
8 drops geranium essential oil

Method

1. Mix all ingredients together in a clean beaker and pour into a bottle.

2. Place the lid onto the bottle and give it a good shake.

3. Label the bottle so you can identify the contents.

Directions for use

Massage the cleanser onto your face. Wipe off using a tissue or cotton-wool pad. Follow by using a suitable toner to remove any traces of the cleanser.

Shelf life

• 12 months

VARIATIONS

As long as you stick to the quantities of oils and emulsifier, you can substitute other ingredients that are more suitable for different skin types. All the variation examples given here follow the same method steps and have the same shelf life as the Total Wipeout Balancing Cleanser on page 69 unless otherwise specified.

GRAPEFRUIT RUSH CLEANSER
For oily skin

50g jojoba oil
25g grapeseed oil
15g castor oil
8g sucragel
8 drops grapefruit essential oil

NEROLI NURTURE SOFTENING CLEANSER
For mature skin

50g apricot kernel oil
25g rice bran oil
1g vitamin E oil
15g castor oil
8g sucragel
8 drops neroli essential oil

Skin-softening Soothing Cleanser
For sensitive skin

50g olive oil
25g rosehip oil
15g castor oil
8g sucragel
8 drops chamomile essential oil

Cleanse & Hydrate Cleanser
For dry skin

50g jojoba oil
20g fractionated coconut oil
20g castor oil
8g sucragel
8 drops rose essential oil

Pore-refiner Cleanser
For problem skin

50g jojoba oil
25g grapeseed oil
15g castor oil
8g sucragel
8 drops patchouli essential oil

Cleansing waters

Cleansing waters are less viscous than cleansing oils, and rather than being massaged onto the face, these are always applied using cotton-wool pads and wiped across the skin. They make very effective cleansers and are light and easy to use.

The sucragel acts as a liquid emulsifier, allowing the oils and waters to mix and reducing any oily feeling on the skin. Since the ingredients may separate in the bottle, cleansing waters should always be shaken before use. I've suggested sucragel as the liquid emulsifier, but you can use polysorbate, sulphonated caster oil or other liquid emulsifiers.

SENSITIVE SKIN HONEY CLEANSING WATER

50g rose water
10g sucragel
15g apricot kernel oil
5g glycerine
5g runny honey
1g preservative (optional)
4 drops rose essential oil
1 drop mandarin essential oil

Method
1. Put all the ingredients in a screwtop bottle and shake to ensure that everything is mixed thoroughly.

2. Label the bottle so that you can identify the contents.

Directions for use
Shake the bottle before use. Place a little of the cleansing water on a cotton-wool pad and wipe over the face in large sweeping movements.

Shelf life
• 6 weeks (without preservative, but a couple of weeks longer if kept in the fridge)
• 12 months (with preservative)

VARIATIONS

Once you're comfortable understanding which ingredients are suitable for different skin types and conditions, you'll be able to create your own versions of these products. In the meantime, here are a few that work well. Both variation examples follow the same method steps and have the same shelf life as the Sensitive Skin Honey Cleansing Water.

PEPPERMINT REFRESHER CLEANSING WATER
For problem skin

40g peppermint water
10g spring water
10g sucragel
15g grapeseed oil
1g preservative (optional)
5 drops rosemary essential oil

COCONUT & LIME CLEANSING WATER
For all skin types

20g orange flower water
30g spring water
10g sucragel
15g fractionated coconut oil
1g preservative (optional)
5 drops lime essential oil

Creamy Cleansers

This is my personal favourite style of cleanser and it's one I use daily. You can use a hot cloth as part of the treatment, or remove the cleanser with tissue or cotton-wool pads. I personally think that gentle rubbing with hot muslin makes this cleanser a real treat to use. It's mild and gentle and literally melts away your make-up.

The cleanser is a blend of water and oil, so it requires an emulsifying ingredient. The oil-and-water emulsion method is used in many cosmetic preparations, including hair conditioners, liquid foundations, moisturisers and body butters. Please see the section on water and oil emulsions (page 158) to understand the principle behind emulsification.

This cleanser is safe and very good at removing mascara, but please make sure you keep your eyes shut when cleaning them to avoid getting the cleanser in your eye. If it does go in your eye, wipe your eye with the muslin to remove the cleanser, then rinse your eye with tepid water until all traces of cleanser have been removed. If an uncomfortable sensation occurs, seek medical help.

ROSY DEW CLEANSER
For dry skin

20g apricot kernel oil
15g castor oil
12g emulsifying wax NF
60g spring water
30g rose water
5g glycerine
1g preservative (optional)
12 drops rose essential oil

Method

1. Weigh the apricot kernel and castor oils and put them in a heatproof container. Add the emulsifying wax and stand the heatproof container in a pan of simmering water.

2. Pour the spring and rose waters into another heatproof container and add the glycerine. Stand this heatproof container in a pan of simmering water. If you wish to use the preservative, add this to the waters container and heat it with the waters and glycerine.

3. Stir the oils container gently every so often until the emulsifying wax has completely melted. Once it has melted, remove both heatproof containers from the heat. Pour the warmed waters and glycerine mix into the oils and stir gently for at least 3 minutes.

4. Leave the mixture to stand for 1 minute, then stir again for 1 minute. Repeat this process a few times while the mixture cools.

5. If the mixture starts to separate, stir a little more briskly to incorporate the oils and waters. If this fails and it still separates, put the heatproof container back into the simmering water and stir until the mixture blends together again. Remove from the heat and stir gently but continuously until the mixture cools (repeat if it separates again). If it continues to separate, add another 1–2g emulsifying wax and melt the wax into the mixture.

6. As the mixture cools, it will become slightly thicker. Once it has cooled to tepid, add the drops of essential oil and continue mixing to ensure thorough distribution of the oil.

7. When the cleanser is cold, place it into your container. Label the container so you can identify the contents.

Directions for use
Massage the cleanser onto your face. Run a muslin cloth under hand-hot water, squeezing out any excess. Rub the cloth in little circular movements on your face. Rinse your face with tepid water and pat dry using a soft clean towel. Rinse the muslin well after use.

Shelf life
• 4 weeks (without preservative)
• 12 months (if using the preservative)

VARIATIONS

There are many ways of varying the creamy cleanser recipe. You can swap oils, waters and essential oils to make the cleanser more suitable for different skin types and conditions. Here are a few suggestions to get you started.

All variation examples follow the same method steps and have the same shelf life as the Rosy Dew Cleanser on pages 74–5 unless otherwise specified.

ORANGE BLOSSOM GENTLE CLEANSER
For mature skin

20g apricot kernel oil
15g castor oil
12g emulsifying wax NF
30g orange flower water
40g spring water
5g glycerine
1g preservative (optional)
12 drops neroli essential oil

NATURAL SKIN CLEANSER
For the most sensitive skin

10g olive oil
10g apricot kernel
15g castor oil
12g emulsifying wax NF
40g rose water
50g spring water
5g glycerine
1g preservative (optional)
12 drops chamomile essential oil

Deep Cleanse & Purify Skin Milk
For problem skin

A deep cleanser for problem skin. The tea tree water, base and essential oils will help prevent infection and reduce inflammation. This cleanser should be applied using four cotton-wool pads. Use a clean pad for each of the following areas: the left cheek, the right cheek, the forehead and the chin and jawbone area.

10g jojoba oil
10g hazelnut oil
5g apricot kernel oil
5g castor oil
14g emulsifying wax NF
50g tea tree water
10g aloe vera
30g spring water
1g preservative (optional)
6 drops eucalyptus essential oil
6 drops rosemary essential oil

Follow the method directions on pages 74–5, but include the aloe vera in the heatproof container with the waters and preservative.

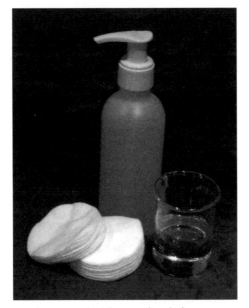

Cleansers can be removed with a muslin cloth or cotton wool pads

OILY SKIN-REFINING CLEANSER

15g grapeseed oil
15g castor oil
12g emulsifying wax NF
50g witch hazel
40g spring water
5g glycerine
1g preservative (optional)
12 drops cedar essential oil

REBALANCER FACIAL CLEANSER
For combination skin

15g jojoba oil
15g castor oil
12g emulsifying wax NF
40g lavender water
40g spring water
5g glycerine
1g preservative (optional)
12 drops geranium essential oil

EXFOLIATING

Exfoliating is the skin's natural act of shedding dead skin cells. This occurs all the time as your body creates new cells in the basal layer of the epidermis and pushes them to the skin's surface. Eventually the dead cells dislodge and fall away. Dead skin cannot absorb moisture, so putting moisturising cream on flaky dead skin will not replenish dead cells.

The act of exfoliating, sloughing off the dead cells by rubbing a slightly abrasive cleanser over your skin, reveals a fresher, newer layer of skin underneath. The rubbing also stimulates circulation, helping the flow of oxygen in the blood, encouraging growth of new cells in the basal layer and speeding their rise to the surface. The benefits are healthy, luminous skin.

How & when to exfoliate

An exfoliating cleanser is a cleanser that has small particles in it. These particles are mildly abrasive and, when rubbed onto the skin, will gently shed dead skin and help to dislodge dry, flaky skin.

An exfoliator's particles should suspend in your cleanser, being equally distributed throughout the product. Natural ingredients used as exfoliating items include crushed nut shells, oats, brown sugar, finely ground salt and coarsely ground bamboo powder.

Apply the exfoliating cleanser either directly to your clean hands or onto a cotton-wool pad or tissue. Gently wipe the cleanser across your face in sweeping movements. Massage the skin gently in tiny circles, paying careful attention to your forehead, sides of the nose and chin areas. Be careful to avoid the eye area completely.

Don't massage too hard. You are supposed to be shifting and dislodging dead skin cells, not scrubbing hard to remove precious skin! The purpose is to leave the skin glowing, translucent and healthily pink.

One you have exfoliated, wipe off residue with a tissue or cotton-wool pad and rinse your face with tepid water. Apply your moisturiser after patting your face dry with a clean towel.

Exfoliating your face in this way should take you approximately four minutes. Ideally you should exfoliate once a week. Those with oily skin can benefit from exfoliating twice a week and those with very dry or sensitive skin should exfoliate every other week.

Exfoliating recipes

In each of these recipes you can choose which exfoliating ingredient you wish to use. How much you use is up to you, too; I've suggested enough to give you a gentle scrub, but it's fine to add up to double the amount indicated.

The recipes are oil and water emulsions that are a little thicker than the oil and water cleansers on pages 74–8. This helps suspend the exfoliating particles so that they don't sink to the bottom of the cleanser.

The recipes are suitable for all skin types. Sensitive skin types should limit the use to once a fortnight; dry, normal and combination skin types can use these once a week, and oily or problem skin types can use these twice weekly.

REPLENISH EXFOLIATING CLEANSER

15g peach kernel oil
15g grapeseed oil
15g emulsifying wax NF
60g spring water
10g glycerine
1g preservative (optional)
6 drops grapefruit essential oil
4 drops eucalyptus essential oil
3g (1 flat teaspoon) exfoliating ingredient (jojoba beads, crushed almond shells or bamboo powder)

Method
1. Weigh the oils and the emulsifying wax and put them in a heatproof container. Stand the heatproof container in a pan of simmering water.

2. Put the waters, glycerine and preservative (if using) in another heatproof container and stand this in a pan of simmering water.

3. Stir the oils container gently every so often until the emulsifying wax has completely melted. Once the wax has melted, remove both heatproof containers from the heat. Pour the warmed waters and glycerine mix into the oils and stir gently for at least 3 minutes.

4. Leave the mixture to stand for 1 minute and then stir again for 1 minute. Repeat this process a few times while the mixture cools.

5. If the mixture starts to separate, stir briskly or put back on the heat source and stir until the liquids have recombined. Remove from the heat and stir while the mixture cools.

6. As the mixture cools, it will become slightly thicker. Once it has cooled to tepid, add the drops of essential oil and continue mixing to ensure thorough distribution of the essential oil.

7. When the cleanser is cold, add your exfoliating ingredient and stir to ensure that it is distributed evenly throughout the cleanser. Put the exfoliating cleanser in a suitable container and label the container so you can identify the contents.

Directions for use
Apply the exfoliating cleanser to your face in gentle sweeping movements using clean hands or a cotton-wool pad or tissue. Gently massage the skin in tiny circles, paying careful attention to the forehead, sides of the nose and chin areas. Avoid the eye area completely, and don't massage too hard.

Wipe off any residue with a tissue or cotton-wool pad and rinse your face with tepid water. Pat your face dry with a clean towel, then apply moisturiser.

Shelf life
• 4 weeks (without preservative)
• 12 months (with preservative)

VARIATIONS

Any of the creamy cleanser recipes on pages 74–8 can be modified to become an exfoliating cleanser. Unless otherwise specified, all variations listed here follow the same method and have the same shelf life as the Replenish Exfoliating Cleanser (pages 80–1).

TRUE GRIT SKIN POLISH

15g sweet almond oil
15g sunflower oil
15g emulsifying wax NF
40g spring water
20g herbal water
10g glycerine
1g preservative (optional)
4 drops rosemary essential oil
4 drops clary sage essential oil
3g (1 flat teaspoon) exfoliating ingredient (jojoba beads, crushed almond shells or bamboo powder)

SWEET SUGAR SCRUB WITH CARROT HEALTHY SKIN POLISH

Carrot oil is particularly nutritious and a rich source of vitamins A, B, C, D, E and F. The oil is made with macerated carrot that has been soaking in a base oil (usually sunflower). It is usually a very bright orange colour and needs to be used sparingly, especially in leave-on products, as it can stain the skin.

15g fractionated coconut oil
10g carrot tissue oil
15g emulsifying wax NF
40g spring water
20g orange flower water
10g glycerine
1g preservative (optional)
4 drops neroli essential oil
4 drops sweet orange essential oil
5g soft brown sugar

Micro-abrasion Skin-softening Cleanser

15g shea butter oil
20g apricot kernel oil
15g emulsifying wax NF
35g lavender water
25g spring water
10g glycerine
1g preservative (optional)
10 drops lavender essential oil
5g bamboo powder

Method

1. Treat the shea butter as an oil and melt it in a heatproof container with the apricot kernel oil and the emulsifying wax.

2. Continue as per the recipe for an oil and water cleanser on pages 80–1.

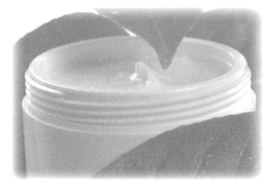

TONING

Toners are used to remove any remaining cleanser and wipe away excess sebum. They close open pores which helps to reduce the chance of bacteria entering the skin. Toners are usually cooling and refreshing.

Many people skip the toning stage during their skincare routine, yet this can be one of the most relaxing and beneficial stages since it can help soothe and balance the pH (skin acidity). The skin's natural pH is 5.5.

How & when to tone

Apply your toner to a pad of cotton wool and wipe it across your face in long, sweeping movements; again, wipe across and up rather than across and down, doing what you can to put off the inevitable skin sag.

Pay careful attention to the crevices either side of your nose, but be careful not to get too close to the eye area. Ensure you pay attention to your hairline, the edges of your face and under your chin as these areas can often be left with traces of cleanser. Your moisturiser will absorb much easier and faster after an application of toner.

Toning your face in this way should take you less than one minute and should be carried out each time you cleanse your face. Toning can also be a refreshing, cooling treatment that can be undertaken on a hot, sticky day without having to cleanse beforehand.

Toner recipes

The toners made in the following recipes can also be used as a cooling and refreshing facial spritz. Instead of packing them in a bottle with screwtop lid, put them in a bottle with a very fine spray attachment, pop them in your handbag and you can have a cool, refreshing moment wherever you are and whenever you need it! If making a facial spritz, consider leaving out the xanthan gum to keep the liquid sufficiently thin and prevent it from blocking the spray mechanism.

If you find xanthan gum a little tricky to use, you can leave it out in any case. Xanthan gum gives a slight viscosity to your toner, which helps it remain on the face before evaporating. It also gives toner a lovely silky feel, allowing it to glide effortlessly across your face. If you can include it, you'll be pleased with the results.

You only need a small quantity of xanthan gum to make a difference. If you feel you have overdone it and your product is too thick, simply add a little more spring water or floral water to the bottle and give it a really good shake to incorporate it.

ORANGE BLOSSOM & GLYCERINE SWEET FACIAL TONIC

A good all-round tonic that will suit all skin types. Use it in the morning, after cleansing and before moisturising to perk up your skin.

35g spring water
3g glycerine
15g aloe vera
40g orange blossom water
0.5g preservative (optional)
5 drops sweet orange essential oil
0.5g xanthan gum*

---

*About ⅕ teaspoon is sufficient for this amount. Use less for a thin, more liquid toner. Don't use any more than 0.5g otherwise you'll be on your way to creating a gel.

Method

1. Pour the spring water in a heatproof jug or bowl and carefully sprinkle the xanthan gum over the top. Stir to dissolve the gum. If the gum collects into little clumps, squash these against the side of the bowl in an effort to disperse them.

2. As it softens in water, xanthan gum will dissolve eventually and simply disappear. Warming the water can speed this process: simply stand the spring water and xanthan gum container in a pan of simmering water and stir fairly briskly until the water has warmed up (don't let it boil; hot-bathwater temperature is sufficient). Remove from the heat and stir until the xanthan gum is dissolved. Don't worry if it isn't fully dissolved; it will continue to soften in the bottle as it absorbs liquid. If you omit the xanthan gum, the spring water can be used cold, straight from the bottle.

3. Put the other ingredients (including the preservative, if using) into a jug or bowl and add the cooled xanthan water, which may well be thickening into a soft gel. Stir to incorporate the ingredients, then pour into a bottle and label.

Directions for use

Best used after cleansing, but it can be used at any time of day to cool and refresh. Shake the bottle before use. Pour a little toner onto cotton wool and wipe over your face in sweeping up and out movements, paying careful attention to the area around your nose. There is no need to rinse this product off.

Shelf life

- 4–5 weeks (without preservative; if possible, keep in the refrigerator)
- 9 months (with preservative)

Variations

Toners can be made using water that you have infused with herbs, flowers and spices. See 'How to make a water infusion', page 136, for more information. Unless otherwise specified, all toner recipes follow the same method and have the same shelf life as the Orange Blossom & Glycerine Sweet Facial Tonic on page 85.

Basking Rose Soothing Toner

The perfect toner for sensitive skin, this toner will help to reduce any redness and soothe inflamed areas while imparting a gorgeous aroma!

30g spring water
0.5g xanthan gum (slightly less is absolutely fine)
10g glycerine
50g rose water
0.5g preservative (optional)
3 drops rose essential oil
2 drops chamomile essential oil

Citrus Pure Toner
for oily skin

Beautifully refreshing! I like to use this as a very light body spray. The clean, fresh uplifting aroma of the lemon and bergamot also helps target oily skin.

50g lemon water
30g bergamot water
0.5g xanthan gum (slightly less is absolutely fine)
15g aloe vera
0.5g preservative (optional)
4 drops lemon essential oil

Rebalancing Facial Tonic

The perfect toner for combination skins. If you don't have rose geranium water, geranium water will give you the same results. The only difference is the aroma, as the rose geranium is more floral than the normal, slightly spicy geranium smell. The rose essential oil will add to the floral aroma as well as helping drier skin areas. Apple cider vinegar helps to readjust any misalignment in the acidity of your skin and restore it to the perfect pH.

25g spring water
0.5g xanthan gum (slightly less is absolutely fine)
4g glycerine
55g rose geranium water
10g ylang-ylang water
5g apple cider vinegar
0.5g preservative (optional)
2 drops rose essential oil
2 drops rose geranium essential oil

Tea Tree Tonic with Mint & Aloe Vera

This toner is useful for a spotty skin, where the spots have are likely to be caused by clogged pores in an oily skin. This also makes a wonderfully cooling foot spray if you omit the xanthan gum.

20g spring water
0.5g xanthan gum (again slightly less is absolutely fine)
5g glycerine
20g aloe vera
35g tea tree water
20g peppermint water
0.5g preservative (optional)
3 drops tea tree essential oil
3 drops lavender essential oil

FRANKINCENSE QUENCHER
for maturing skin

This is especially good when used in the evenings. Frankincense is used in meditation and will help you to relax before sleeping. I've included a drop of carrot seed oil in the toner as this is one of the best essential oils for rejuvenating skin. It has a slightly earthy aroma which isn't to everyone's taste, but the frankincense water and oil will help to mask the smell.

Don't confuse carrot seed essential oil, made by steam-distilling the seeds of the carrot, with carrot tissue oil, which is the carrot vegetable infused in a base oil. Both are wonderful additions to skincare products, but are very different to each other.

30g spring water
0.5g xanthan gum (slightly less is absolutely fine)
5g glycerine
60g frankincense water
0.5g preservative (optional)
4 drops frankincense essential oil
1 drops carrot seed essential oil

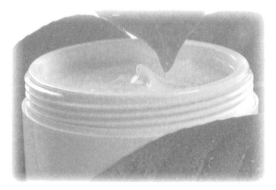

MOISTURISING

Moisturising is probably the most prevalent skincare routine worldwide. It is a key process because it helps to lock in the skin's natural moisture and retain its natural suppleness and flexibility.

A moisturiser will rehydrate your skin and help create a protective barrier against air pollution and other possible environmental damage. A good moisturiser will penetrate the epidermis and keep your skin lithe and supple all day. Moisturising is a necessity, whether you wear make-up or not.

How & when to moisturise

Apply your moisturiser to a clean, toned face. Put your moisturiser on with clean fingertips, rubbing the moisturiser onto your skin gently, following the contours of your face. Never drag the skin, but use light, feathery strokes. Gently massage with your fingertips in small, circular movements and allow the moisturiser to sink in before applying your make-up.

You can use a richer moisturiser at night, or apply a more generous helping of your daytime moisturiser. You should always moisturise every morning before applying your make-up and every night after removing your make-up.

Moisturise more frequently if you have a dry skin. Moisturising regularly will help you to reap the rewards of having a lovely, healthy-looking skin and delay signs of aging.

Moisturising your face as described should take you approximately two minutes, but do allow some extra time for the moisturiser to sink in before applying make-up.

Moisturising cream recipes

Making your own moisturising products is where you can make a big difference to your skin. Many of the commercially prepared creams contain fillers to bulk out the products, and specialist ingredients that temporarily make your skin look and feel lovely but have no long-lasting effects.

In contrast, the recipes for the creams given in the next few pages guarantee a boost of moisture, helping your skin not only right now, but also well into the future. Think of these creams as the perfect nutritional diet for your skin.

24-hour Moisture Boost

For dry skin

The three oils used in this recipe have been selected for their wonderful hydrating properties. Not only will this moisturising cream feel wonderful on your skin, but it will also continue to keep your skin moisturised throughout the day.

Avocado oil is one of my favourite oils and it is one that I carry around with me. It is light enough to be applied directly onto the skin without leaving any greasy residue. Rich and penetrating, avocado oil comes from the flesh of the avocado and is a natural source of vitamins A and D and betacarotene. The plant steroids in the oil help soften the skin, making it a super-hydrating oil.

Argan oil is probably the most expensive oil we use at Plush Folly. A very rich source of vitamin E and antioxidants, argan oil is considered a luxury oil in skincare treatments and is very nourishing, healing and anti-aging. It has a natural moisturising effect and will continue to hydrate the skin long after it is applied.

Kukui nut oil is rich in essential fatty acids and easily absorbed by the skin. The oil will help to soften, smooth, moisturise and renew dry, mature and problem skin. It penetrates the skin well and helps improve its ability to retain moisture.

These three oils used together make one very special moisturising cream.

15g avocado oil
10g argan oil
10g kukui nut oil
14g emulsifying wax NF
30g orange flower water
30g spring water
1g preservative (optional)
2 drops myrrh essential oil
6 drops neroli essential oil

Method

1. The procedure is the same as described in the oil and water emulsion method as used in the hot-cloth cleanser recipes on page 67. Put the oils and the emulsifying wax in a heatproof jug or bowl and stand it in a pan of simmering water, stirring gently every so often to help the wax melt.

2. Put the waters and preservative (if using) in a heatproof jug or bowl and stand this in a pan of simmering water, too. Heat the waters, but don't allow them to boil.

3. Once the emulsifying wax has melted, remove both heatproof containers from the heat. Pour the warmed waters into the oils and stir gently for at least 3 minutes.

4. Leave the mixture to stand for 1 minute and then stir again for 1 minute. Repeat this process a few times while the mixture cools.

5. If the mixture starts to separate, stir a little more briskly to incorporate the oils and waters. If this fails and it still separates, put the heatproof container back into the simmering water and stir until the mixture blends together again. Remove from the heat and stir gently but continuously until the mixture cools down (repeat if it separates again). If it continues to separate, add another 1–2g emulsifying wax and melt the wax into the mixture.

6. As the mixture cools, it will become slightly thicker. Add the drops of essential oil once it has started to thicken. Continue mixing to ensure their thorough distribution.

7. Put the moisturiser into your container. Label the container so you can identify the contents.

Directions for use

Scoop a little moisturiser onto your clean fingers and place a little blob on each cheek, your chin, nose and forehead. Gently extend the little blobs so that the entire face is covered by gently massaging the cream into your skin.

Shelf life
- 4 weeks (without preservative)
- 12 months (with preservative)

VARIATIONS

There are so many base oils to choose from that varying the recipe to suit other skin types is infinitely possible. As well as changing the oils, consider changing the floral water and the essential oils using the appropriate charts in this book. You can increase the quantity of water to make a runnier cream or lotion, or reduce the amount of water to make a much thicker, richer cream. Unless otherwise specified, all variations given here follow the same method steps and have the same shelf life as the 24-hour Moisture Boost on pages 90–1.

PERFECT SKIN CREAM

For oily skin

If you have oily skin, then here is something to celebrate! Oily skin types tend to develop the signs of aging skin far slower than those with dry skin. The skin's natural sebum lubricates the skin, keeping it flexible and supple, which delays the appearance of fine lines and wrinkles.
This cleanser will ensure that excess sebum is mopped up and pores are kept clean and clear. The lemon is astringent and will help to close the pores, while the juniper berry and grapefruit oils do their best to unclog. The base oils selected will help to refine and tone, leaving your skin looking clean, clear and bright.

10g walnut oil
15g cherry kernel oil
12g emulsifying wax NF
20g lemon grass water
40g spring water
1g preservative (optional)
2 drops grapefruit essential oil
3 drops lemon essential oil
2 drops juniper berry essential oil

Radiance Moisture

For combination skin

Essential oils of ylang-ylang and sandalwood help control and rebalance overly dry or oily patches. To hydrate I have selected jojoba oil for its ability to trick the sebaceous glands into producing precise quantities of sebum, while ensuring that the skin is kept moisturised and supple. Melon seed oil has been included for its ultra-quick absorbing ability and wonderful wealth of omegas 3 and 6, and I've added a little wheatgerm oil to help sooth, hydrate and boost the vitamin E content.

15g melon seed oil
15g jojoba oil
5g wheatgerm oil
14g emulsifying wax NF
30g lavender water
30g spring water
1g preservative (optional)
2 drops sandalwood essential oil
6 drops ylang-ylang essential oil

Repair & Purify

For problem skin

A hydrating cream that is clever enough to treat rashes and spots and soothe sore and inflamed areas. The rosehip oil breaks down any scar tissue and helps restore the skin to its former, healthy state. Essential oils of eucalyptus, bergamot and petitgrain support the healing properties of the base oils, as well as offering anti-inflammatory and decongesting abilities.

14g avocado oil
10g rosehip oil
1g vitamin E
10g emulsifying wax NF
30g bergamot water
30g spring water
1g preservative (optional)
2 drops eucalyptus essential oil
3 drops petitgrain essential oil
2 drops bergamot essential oil

Dew Soft Intense Moisture
For sensitive skin

A super-hydrating skin-softening cream that is so gentle it makes a perfect treatment for sensitive skin types. The combination of apricot kernel, safflower and rosehip oils makes this cream softening, soothing and calming, while the essential oils of rose and rosewood ensure hydration and calming of any inflamed or itchy areas.

5g apricot kernel oil
10g rosehip oil
15g safflower oil
14g emulsifying wax NF
20g rose water
40g spring water
1g preservative (optional)
4 drops rose essential oil
3 drops rosewood essential oil

Rose & Frankincense Deep Moisture
For mature skin

For the perfect anti-aging cream, I have teamed up avocado with evening primrose oil. I've also included vitamin E so that this cream will help fade age spots, reduce sun damage and scarring. The avocado and evening primrose oils target wrinkles and encourage the growth of new skin. The delightfully aromatic blend of frankincense and rose ensure that this moisturising cream hydrates and softens while boosting the effectiveness of skin-cell regeneration from the base oils. An absolutely fabulous cream.

15g avocado oil
10g evening primrose oil
1g vitamin E oil
15g emulsifying wax NF
40g rose water
20g spring water
1g preservative (optional)
4 drops frankincense essential oil
3 drops rose essential oil

Night creams

Night creams are intense treatments designed to be applied to the skin last thing before you retire to bed. They should be sufficiently formulated so that they keep working into, and through, the night without being rubbed off on your pillow. I love the idea of the ingredients working hard to treat my face while I sleep! Note: all night-cream recipes have the same shelf life as Sleep Easy Face Treat.

SLEEP EASY FACE TREAT

Jasmine essential oil promotes a peaceful sleep, while the oils, butters and beeswax soften, hydrate and work wonders on skin. Massage a little of this into your face after cleansing and toning.

10g evening primrose oil
10g shea butter
10g emulsifying wax NF
5g beeswax
30g rose water
0.5g preservative (optional)
10g rosehip oil
8 drops jasmine essential oil

Method
1. Put the evening primrose oil, shea butter and waxes in a heatproof jug or bowl. Stand it in a pan of simmering water, stirring gently every so often to help the waxes melt.

2. Put the rose water and preservative (if using) in a heatproof jug or bowl and stand this in a pan of simmering water, too, until it is hand-hot.

3. Once the waxes have melted, remove both heatproof containers from the heat. Pour the warmed waters into the oils and stir gently for at least 3 minutes. Add the rosehip oil and stir again. Leave the mixture to stand for 1 minute and then stir again for 1 minute. Add the jasmine essential oil and stir again.

4. Once the mixture has cooled and thickened, put it into a suitable container. Label the container so that you can identify its contents.

Shelf life
• 4 weeks (without preservative)
• 12 months (with preservative)

Radiance Night Cream

The restorative, rejuvenating oils help repair and revive your skin while you sleep.

10g shea butter
10g emulsifying wax NF
5g beeswax
5g sunflower oil
30g orange blossom water
0.5g preservative (optional)
4 drops bergamot essential oil
4 drops carrot seed oil
10g hemp seed oil
5g rosehip oil

Method

Use the same method for the Sleep Easy Face Treat on page 95, but don't heat the hemp or rosehip oils. Add these to the mixture once the oils, butters, waxes and waters have been combined.

Hydration Smoother Night Slumber Cream

A hydrating night cream that will help soften skin and smooth uneven skin texture.

10g calendula oil
10g wheatgerm oil
10g cocoa butter
12g emulsifying wax NF
0.5g preservative (optional)
4 drops rose essential oil
4 drops frankincense essential oil

Method

Use the same method for the Sleep Easy Face Treat on page 95.

Intensive Night Cream

This ultra-moisturising cream helps to soothe and calm any sore, inflamed areas while firming and improving elasticity.

10g mango butter
5g shea butter
5g grapeseed oil
5g jojoba oil
10g emulsifying wax NF
30g rose water
20g orange blossom water
0.5 preservative (optional)
2 drops patchouli essential oil
4 drops sweet orange essential oil
5g flaxseed oil

Method

Use the same method for the Sleep Easy Face Treat on page 95, but reserve the flaxseed oil and add it once the butters, oils, wax and waters have been combined.

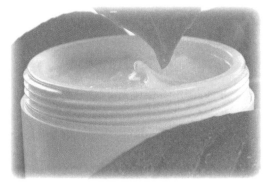

SPECIALIST TREATMENTS

Specialist treatments are designed help target a particular skin problem or to give your skin a nourishing boost.

Detoxing your skin using a face mask

A detox treatment will help remove impurities on and in the top layers of your skin, rid the skin of toxins and boost cell renewal. The most common detox treatment is to deep-cleanse using a clay face mask, which will help draw out dirt and grime from the top layers of the epidermis. Face masks can also help stimulate circulation and nourish your skin with extra vitamins and minerals.

Additionally, a face mask assists the skin by helping to shed dead cells and unblocking pores. This, in turn, will help your cleansing, toning and moisturising products work more effectively. A face mask can give you an immediate beauty boost and make your skin look instantly radiant, glowing and healthy.

Some face masks may also contain ingredients that will help feed and nourish your skin. Ingredients that may be added include dairy powders (for softening the skin), fruit powders (for natural fruit acids and vitamins), seaweed (for trace elements and minerals) and oils (for nourishing and maintaining levels of moisture). To summarize then, face masks help your skin by:

- Absorbing excess oils, drawing out toxins and impurities;
- Gently exfoliating;
- Deep cleansing;
- Balancing and moisturising;
- Helping to even out skin tone;
- Treating blackheads, pimples and other blemishes; and
- Conditioning and refining.

While face masks all share a similar function, they come in many different styles. Clay masks are designed to set hard and make your face feel taught. Gel masks are designed to be cool and soothing, and some masks are designed to peel off, removing dirt and flakes as if you are shedding your skin. Other masks are designed to nourish, moisturise and encourage cell renewal.

How & when to use a face mask

Skin can react to face masks in different ways, and the surge of intensive treatment can sometimes make your skin actually look worse shortly afterwards. This isn't necessarily a bad sign, though, because it may indicate that congested toxins and impurities have come to the surface and are being eliminated. However, avoid using a face mask a day or two before a big event just in case your skin decides to erupt on you. Please remember to do a patch test before use if you're uncertain of the suitability of any cosmetic product.

To use a face mask, first tie your hair back and clip up any that may fall onto your face. Remove all traces of make-up and apply the face mask to clean skin.

Place some of the mask onto your clean fingertips or a soft brush and carefully apply to your face in a consistent layer, using small, sweeping movements. Do not make the layer too thick, as it may be too heavy and attempt to slip off rather than dry on your skin. Avoid putting the face mask on your eye and lip areas. Applying a little lip balm before applying the face mask helps protect your lips.

Once you're happy with the coverage, wash your hands and lie or sit somewhere quietly while the mask does its magic.

Once the allotted time has gone by, remove the mask, depending on its type. If your face mask is the type that doesn't set hard, this can be wiped off and any traces removed with a cleanser. The easiest way to remove a mask that has gone hard is to lean over the basin (or do this in the bath), grimace and pull faces by opening your mouth as wide as you can and then pulling it taught as if you are blowing one very long k-i-s-s. Make your face look as surprised as it can be and then 'collapse' your face as if you were playing the part of a very old woman in a pantomime. Not only is this a fabulous workout for your facial muscles, but it also helps loosen the face mask so that it begins to crack and crumble off.

Depending on how well your face mask has adhered to your face, you can remove the bulk of it by rubbing it in very fine, small circles on your skin. This also helps remove dead skin cells and flaky patches. When you're happy that you've removed all that you can in this way, simply rinse the rest off in tepid water.

Always apply a moisturiser after you have used a face mask and drink a glass of water.

Depending on your skin type and the style of face mask you use, a face mask treatment should be limited to once a week, or even less frequently. Dry, mature and sensitive skins require a more gentle face mask than combination, normal and problem skins.

Face mask recipes

The face masks can be used on all skin types by varying the clay colour. I've selected six of my favourite masks and substituted the clays so there is a mask for each skin type. Mix and match the ingredients in the recipes to make one that's perfect for you.

Guidelines for clay suitability	
Green Clay	Normal / Oily Skin
Red Clay	Normal Skin
White Clay	Normal / Combination / Sensitive Skin
Pink Clay	Dry / Sensitive Skin
Yellow Clay	Normal / Oily Skin
Fuller's Earth	Normal / Oily Skin

Clays are dried naturally in the sun and are intensely rich in minerals such as oxides, magnesium, calcium, potassium, dolomite, silica, manganese, phosphorous, silicon, copper and selenium. Clay will draw out impurities and soak up excess oiliness. If your skin is dry to begin with, you may find that a clay mask requires the addition of a little oil to keep it from being too drying.

Unless otherwise specified, all face-mask recipes have the same shelf life as the Deep Down & Dirty Mineral Mud Mask.

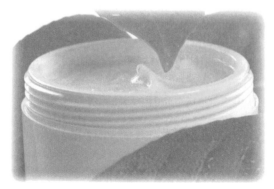

Deep Down & Dirty Mineral Mud Mask

For oily skin

Dead Sea mud improves circulation, deep-cleanses and detoxifies, softens and relieves itchiness, so it makes a marvellous addition to any face mask. It can be used on its own without the addition of clay, but many skins find this a little too strong.

15g white clay
10g fuller's earth
5g Dead Sea mud
30g spring water
0.5g preservative (optional)
4 drops petitgrain
4 drops lemon grass

Method

1. Put the water and preservative (if using) into a bowl. Sprinkle the clay, fuller's earth and Dead Sea mud onto the water and leave to settle. Do not stir for at least 2 minutes while the water absorbs some of the clay powders.

2. After 2 minutes, when you can see that the powders have started to be absorbed into the water, stir gently until thoroughly mixed, stirring and squashing any clumps of powder that may have formed. Add the essential oils and stir again.

3. You may find that the consistency of your face mask is too runny and thin, or too thick and stiff. Each clay absorbs water, and different-coloured clays have different abilities to absorb. To adjust the consistency to suit, add more water or more clay a little at a time until you have reached your desired consistency. The consistency you're looking for is similar to a glossy butter frosting on a cake – thick enough to stand up and hold its shape, but soft enough to be able to spread across your face easily without dripping off.

4. Put your face mask in a container or bag and label it so that you can identify the contents.

Directions for use

1. Thoroughly cleanse your face to remove all traces of make-up. Tie your hair back and away from your face. Moisturise your lips with a little lip balm before applying the mask around the mouth area as this will help prevent the mask from getting on your lips – it doesn't taste nice and may dry them out.

2. Using a brush or very clean fingers, apply a layer of mask onto your face, avoiding the eye area.

3. Leave the mask on until it sets hard. How long this takes depends on how thick a layer you applied and how moist your face is, but allow 15–20 minutes.

4. To remove, stretch your mouth open very wide before removing the mask as this will help remove dead skin cells. Grimace, make on 'O' shape with your mouth, pretend to yawn and generally contort your face into shapes. Once the mask has loosened a little from the skin, either wash off or gently rub the mask in small circular movements to loosen it further, then wash the traces of mask off.

Shelf life
• 2 weeks (without preservative; slightly longer if you keep it in the refrigerator)
• 6 months (with preservative, but make sure the mask is kept airtight so that it doesn't dry out)

PEACHES & CREAM FACE FIX
For sensitive skin

This is so skin-softening that your skin will thank you for it. Buttermilk powder smooths and softens the skin while the addition of peach kernel oil ensures that the mask helps replenish and moisturise, which assists in keeping skin supple. Don't add too much peach kernel oil, as it may not mix with the water and cause your mask to curdle. If this happens, drain away any unwanted water seepage. The mask may not look as pretty as usual, but it will still be fine for use.

15g pink clay
15g white clay
28g spring water
0.5g preservative (optional)
3g peach kernel oil
1 drop carrot seed oil
4 drops rose essential oil

Method
Make the mask up with the clays, preservative (optional) and water as per the recipe on page 101. Add the peach kernel and carrot seed oil with the essential oil; mix well.

Milk & Honey Face Ambrosia
For mature skin

You can add honey powder or runny honey to this mask. Adding runny honey will give a thinner consistency, so you may need to adjust the clay a little to compensate. Add the runny honey after mixing the clay with the water and add the honey powder with the clay.

Honey is a natural humectant, meaning that it attracts moisture from the air and locks it onto its surface. This will ensure that your honey mask will be hydrating as well as deep cleansing. Honey also softens and nourishes the skin.

The essential oils have been selected for their ability to improve collagen formation and skin elasticity and also because they work well with the honey to produce a sweet, aromatic ambrosia.

25g white clay
5g milk powder (full-fat or semi-skimmed)
5g honey powder or 5g runny honey
30g spring water
0.5g preservative (optional)
3 drops sweet orange essential oil
3 drops neroli essential oil
1 drop ylang-ylang

Method

Make the mask up as per the recipe on page 101, add the essential oils and mix well. If the milk powder is a little coarse, grind it down using a pestle and mortar to make it a finer powder.

Dairy Maiden Skin Beauty

For dry skin

This gentle mask's skin-softening ability is boosted by natural yoghurt. Yoghurt is thicker than water so I've cut back on the clay, but you may need to adjust it depending on the thickness of yoghurt used. Rose essential oil with a dash of patchouli helps keep skin clear and bright. Because of the fresh yoghurt, this mask should be used within 2–3 days and must be kept in the fridge, so I've made quantities sufficient for 1–2 masks. For a larger batch to use over a number of weeks, double or treble the recipe quantities, exchange the yoghurt for water and add 0.5–1g preservative.

11g pink clay
5g buttermilk powder
15g natural yoghurt
4g jojoba oil
3 drops rose essential oil
1 drop patchouli essential oil

Method

Make the mask up as per the recipe on page 101. Add the jojoba oil with the essential oils once the powders and waters have been successfully mixed.

Shelf life

• 2–3 days (this mask must be kept in the refrigerator)

Enzyme Fruit Mask
For problem skin

Powdered fruit gives a mask the amino acid, vitamin and enzyme benefits of fresh fruit but with a longer shelf life – providing you use a preservative. Red clay tends to create a thinner, runnier mask, so I've adjusted the liquid content, but play around with the recipe until you find a consistency you like. Zinc oxide helps treat rashes and sore patches and witch hazel has astringent, anti-inflammatory qualities.

20g red clay
5g white clay
2g zinc oxide
5g strawberry powder
10g spring water
8g witch hazel
0.5g preservative (optional)
8 drops sweet orange essential oil

Method
Make the mask as on page 101, adding in the witch hazel with the essential oil.

Double G Marine Vitality Facial Detox Treatment
For combination skins

Rich in minerals, dried seaweed nourishes skin. Its aroma isn't unpleasant, but be sure your essential oils work with it as you'll have this on your face. Grapefruit and geranium oils flush out toxins, plus their refreshing aroma controls the seaweed scent.

20g green clay
5g fuller's earth
5g dried kelp or spirulina
25g spring water
0.5g preservative (optional)
5g jojoba oil
4 drops grapefruit essential oil
5 drops geranium essential oil

Method
Make the mask as on page 101. Add the jojoba oil with the essential oils once the powders and waters have been successfully mixed.

TREATING YOUR SKIN USING A BEAUTÉ GEL

Stress has a great (and usually negative) impact on skin. While skincare products can't eliminate the stresses in your life, they can help soothe your skin and encourage you to slow down and relax for a while. A cooling beauté gel is therapeutic in that it is soothing, calming and helps reduce any inflammation.

A gel treatment is typically made up of water and a gelling ingredient such as xanthan gum, guar or carrageen. On their own, these products would feel cool and refreshing but wouldn't offer any further skincare benefits. However, since the beauté gel treatment is going to be on your skin for 15 minutes or so, the gel can be used as a carrier for other specialist ingredients, allowing them time to sit on your skin while they go to work softening, repairing, toning or smoothing.

A beauté gel is a much softer face mask with added xanthan gum to prevent it from setting hard. For those that don't enjoy the feeling of a tight, unmovable, rock-hard face mask, beauté gels are flexible and lighter.

Using a beauté gel treatment

Take a little beauté gel onto the tip of a clean finger and gently spread or pat the gel on the area you are targeting, being careful to avoid contact with your eyes. Leave the gel on your face for 10–15 minutes.

Depending on the thickness of the gel layer you applied, it may set slightly as it cools and refreshes your skin. To remove, wipe away the gel with tissues, rinse with clean, tepid water and pat dry with a towel. You can use a toner to remove final traces of the gel.

Beauté gel recipes

Depending on the active ingredients in each gel treatment, it may be used as regularly as once a day.

BELLE BELLE BEAUTÉ GEL

This mask will replenish your skin with the addition of jojoba and vitamin E oils, rejuvenate it with the addition of patchouli essential oil and renew it with a little helping of collagen-forming sweet orange.

Enough clay is included to create a paste, and it will be gloopy, reminiscent of wallpaper glue – but don't let that put you off! Beauté gel treatments are cooling, refreshing and a relaxing treat. If you prefer a thinner product, use more water than stated in the recipe. Using less water will make your gel thicker and more paste-like in appearance, but if you can still spread it on your skin, then it will work!

35g spring water
0.5g preservative (optional)
1g xanthan gum
5g jojoba oil
1g vitamin E oil
4 drops sweet orange essential oil
2 drops patchouli essential oil
5g pink clay

Method

1. Put the water and preservative (optional) in a bowl (a breakfast cereal bowl is the ideal size) and sprinkle the xanthan gum over the top. Leave to stand without stirring for 3 minutes.

2. Stir the xanthan gum into the water, mixing as well as you can to break down any lumps. Drizzle in the oils a little at a time, stirring well in between each addition. Add the essential oils and stir again. Add the clay, then give it a brisk stir again. The mixture may look as though it is curdling, but with more mixing, it will come together.

3. Put into a container and label it so that you can identify the contents.

Directions for use

Remove all traces of make-up and tie your hair back off your face. Spread the beauté gel over your face and lie down somewhere for 15–20 minutes while the gel works on your skin. Wipe the beauté gel away with tissues and rinse off any residue.

Shelf life

• 4 weeks (without preservative; this must be kept in the refrigerator)
• 6 months (with preservative and kept in an airtight container)

VARIATIONS

The Belle Belle Beauté Gel recipe on page 107 is completely tailorable. Apart from the xanthan gum, which is needed to create the gel consistency, the ingredients can be swapped around as you think fit. Any oil can be added to replace the jojoba and vitamin E blend. You can add more oil, too, but be prepared for some hefty stirring to prevent the mixture from splitting.

Floral waters or infusions can be used to replace all or some of the water, and the clay can be substituted with dairy or fruit powders, or Dead Sea mud – or be left out entirely. Unless otherwise specified, all beauté gel recipes given here follow the same method steps and have the same shelf life as the Belle Belle Beauté Gel.

TONED TONIC GOLDEN BEAUTÉ GEL

With frankincense and myrrh

While this is the perfect face mask for a dry, tired, dull complexion, it can also be applied to areas of your body as a general treatment tonic. This beauté gel contains no clay, but I have included a little gold mica instead to play along with the gold, frankincense and myrrh theme. The mica brings no active properties, just visual beauty, giving your gel a golden shimmer.

45g spring water
5g grapeseed oil
1g xanthan gum
A pinch of gold mica
0.5g preservative (optional)
5 drops frankincense oil
3 drops myrrh essential oil

CLEAR & BRIGHT EYE GEL

Use the treatment as regularly as once a day to calm tired eyes and reduce puffiness.

2g aloe vera
15g orange flower water
0.5g xanthan gum
20g spring water
0.5g preservative (optional)

Method

1. Add the aloe vera to the water and then mix with the xanthan gum. As this is going on the delicate eye area, I haven't included an essential oil because the flower water and aloe vera will be sufficient as a treatment.

2. To apply your eye gel, take a little gel onto the tip of a clean finger and gently pat it around the eye area, being careful to avoid direct contact with your eyes. Remove after 15 minutes.

DETOX FACIAL TREAT

Use this beauté gel when you've overindulged a little and need to feel that you're doing something to move on from sluggish to energised.

45g spring water
5g hemp seed oil
1g xanthan gum
0.5g preservative (optional)
3 drops bergamot essential oil
2 drops grapefruit essential oil
1 drop carrot seed oil

Vitamin Feed Face Beauté Gel

This is the ultimate pre-party face food! Use this treatment a couple of hours before you get ready to go out partying and enjoy a natural, healthy, good-looking glow. If you want to sparkle, add a tiny amount of cosmetic glitter to the beauté gel to get you in the mood.

35g spring water
10g apple juice
5g avocado oil
1g xanthan gum
A pinch of cosmetic grade glitter (optional)
0.5g preservative (optional)
3 drops rosewood essential oil
2 drops neroli essential oil
1 drop juniper berry oil

Glitter Gel

You can always make up a pot of glitter gel by combining 50g spring water with 0.5g xanthan gum and 0.5g preservative. Add glitter and mix well. Pat a tiny amount of the gel onto skin or into hair and sparkle away!

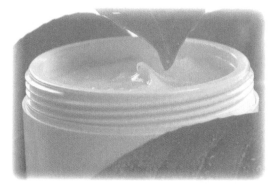

REHYDRATING YOUR SKIN USING A BALM

A skin balm, also known as a salve or ointment, is designed as a huge hydrating boost for parched and very dry skin patches. Although it penetrates the skin and helps to hydrate, a balm doesn't soak into skin completely. Instead, it rests on the surface, locking in moisture and creating a protective barrier between the skin and the air.

A balm should be light enough to allow your skin to breathe, but not as light as a moisturiser. It is therefore generally used on dry skin areas or lips rather than all over the face.

When & how to use a balm

Like a moisturiser, a balm is applied directly to the skin using clean fingers. Instead of spreading the balm across the entire area of your face, carefully massage the area to be treated with a little balm, making sure that you don't agitate the skin unnecessarily.

Depending on the severity of the dry skin area in question, a balm can be applied several times during the day.

Balm recipes

A balm is one of the most flexible products you can make. Although the balms in these recipes are designed to be rubbed onto areas of your face, you can use a balm on other parts of your body. You can easily convert a balm to be a product suitable for:

- hair (as a pre-shampoo treatment or a frizzy ends tamer);
- face (a gentle eye treatment or as a post-cold, flaky-nose salve);
- lip balm (everyone needs one of these);
- arms (to soften those lizard elbows);
- nails (great nail and cuticle treatment);
- hands (a post gardening balm to soothe scratches and blisters);
- chest (chesty rub);
- bottom (on babies – with added zinc to soothe nappy rash);
- legs (super-moisturising, especially scaly shins and knees);
- ankles (useful as an anti-mosquito balm);
- feet (fabulous post-marathon foot therapy, even if you've only run for the bus);
- pulse points (as a solid perfume);
- temples (as an anti-stress, calming two-minute treatment); and
- anywhere (I used to keep a tin of 'Mummy's Magic' in my handbag. It was a great cure-all when the children had bumps, scrapes and grazes).

That's 14 treatments by just varying one recipe!

Basic Beauty Balm

The basic beauty balm is a balm that will help hydrate flaky, dry areas and treat lips. This is the simplest of the balms, but very effective.

5g shea butter
5g cocoa butter
5g olive oil
10g sweet almond oil
5g beeswax
8 drops rose essential oil

Method

1. Put the butters, olive and sweet almond oils and beeswax into a heatproof bowl and stand the bowl in a pan of simmering water. Allow the wax and butters to melt slowly.

2. Once the mixture has melted, remove from the heat and allow to cool a little. Add the rose essential oil and stir well.

3. Pour the mixture into a lidded container, but don't put the lid on until it has cooled sufficiently and formed a solid skin across the surface. Once you can see the skin has formed, or it feels solid to touch, put the lid on. Label the container so that you can identify the contents. Leaving the lid off until the balm is cool and firm prevents any build-up of evaporation in the container.

Directions for use

Rub a little of the balm onto the dry area.

Shelf life

• 18 months

This product does not require a preservative because it doesn't contain any water. See the section on preservatives (page 164) for more information.

Variations

This product is completely flexible. Not only can the ingredients be changed very easily, but the texture and hardness of the final balm can be manipulated, too. An unscented balm is likely to be made up of three different sets of ingredients – butter, wax and base oil. The function of the wax is to add hardness to the balm, while the butters and oils will hydrate.

The Basic Beauty Balm calls for 5g wax, 10g butters and 15g oils. If the proportions are changed to 2g wax, 10g butters and 15g oils, you have a very similar product, but it will be a little softer. A softer balm will be easier to get out of the container – by simply stroking your finger across the surface of the product, a good quantity of balm will transfer.

Using waxes in balms

If you wanted to make a lip balm and pack it in a lip balm tube, a softer balm wouldn't be suitable. A lip balm tube requires a harder balm that can be twisted up and down inside, and rubbed on the lips without risk of it being too soft to wind back down into the container. You would need to increase the beeswax in the lip balm recipe to make sure you had a more solid balm.

Adding too much wax can be a problem, though, because too much wax can make a product too hard and brittle. Wax also shrinks as it cools, causing little holes or cracks to appear in the balm.

Beeswax is a product created by honeybees and as such, may not be included in products suitable for vegans. Waxes such as jojoba and olive wax make suitable alternatives. They work in the same way to harden balms, but don't have the anti-itch, anti-inflammatory, skin-softening and moisture-retaining properties found in beeswax.

Using butters in balms

Rather than increase the amount of wax to make a product harder, consider altering the quantity and style of the butters in the recipe. The Basic Beauty Balm used equal proportions of shea and cocoa butter. Cocoa butter is harder than shea butter, so in order to harden a product you could reduce the amount of shea butter and increase the amount of cocoa butter. For example, the Basic Beauty Balm used 5g shea butter and 5g cocoa butter, making a total of 10g.

If you used 3g shea butter and 7g cocoa butter, you'd have the same amount of butter, but the end product would be harder. Of course, there are many other butters available, too; while cocoa butter is the hardest of them all, there are plenty of butters that are softer than shea butter. So you can see, you can have endless fun playing around with the waxes and the butters to change the consistency of the balms.

Using oils in balms

While changing the type of base oil used in the recipe won't change the final texture or consistency (unless you change the quantity), you can use different base oils to bring different properties to your balm. For example, a balm rich in rosehip oil will help break down and repair scar tissue; a balm with a high castor oil content will create a protective barrier on the skin; and a balm with a high quantity of flaxseed will help to treat any inflamed, dry and itchy areas.

Using essential oils in balms

Essential oils have active properties, and as such can make your balm recipe even more flexible and useful. Looking at the Basic Beauty Balm recipe again, I've included rose essential oil as it is very suitable for dry skin. If you substituted peppermint essential oil for the rose essential oil, this balm would instantly become highly suitable for feet. The balm will work on softening the skin and hydrating hard, cracked skin while the peppermint is cooling, refreshing and deodorising – the perfect treatment after having been on your feet all day.

Similarly, if you use the Basic Beauty Balm and add mandarin and neroli instead of the rose, you instantly have a nail and cuticle treatment. Mandarin and neroli work together to strengthen nails and soften cuticles. Apply this to your nails and fingertips every day for a week and your nails will grow strong and stop splitting.

Changing a balm's texture

Just when you thought you'd covered everything to do with formulating balms, I have one more option to tell you about: whisking your balm. You can change the final texture of your balm by beating the melted mixture as it sets, rather than just melting, mixing and pouring into the container. To achieve this, melt the wax, soften or melt the butters and mix them together in a jug. Add the oils, then beat the mixture with a hand-held whisk until it is light and fluffy.

Leave the mixture to rest for 2 minutes, then beat again for 30 seconds or so. Repeat this process 4–5 times until the balm is creamy, light and fluffy. Add your chosen essential oils and give the balm one more 30-second blitz.

Put the whipped balm into a lidded container and label it so that you can identify the contents.

All balm recipes given here can be either whipped or not, depending on personal preference. Unless otherwise specified, all follow the same method and have the same shelf life as the Basic Beauty Balm on page 112.

Skin-booster Balm

The ingredients in this balm have been chosen for their ability to hydrate deeply and provide moisture over a number of hours.

5g beeswax
15g mango butter
5g cocoa butter
15g jojoba oil
10g sunflower oil
8 drops sandalwood essential oil
4 drops carrot seed essential oil

There There Salve

This is a variation on 'Mummy's Magic'. It is soothing, healing and very restorative.

15g jojoba oil
5g wheatgerm oil
5g rosehip oil
10g mango butter
5g cocoa butter
6g olive wax
1g vitamin E oil
10 drops orange essential oil
4 drops chamomile essential oil

Method
1. Melt the first six ingredients together.

2. Add the vitamin E and essential oils once the balm is off the heat and cooling.

TRIPLE-WHIPPED HEALING BALM

The ingredients in this balm have been chosen for their soothing and healing properties. This balm is whipped to make it lighter, allowing the zinc to be carried in the balm rather than sinking to the bottom, which it is likely to do if the melted balm is mixed with the zinc and then poured straight into the container.

40g shea butter
12g beeswax
20g olive oil
10g zinc oxide
10g borage oil
20g calendula oil
15 drops lavender essential oil
8 drops bergamot essential oil

Method

1. Melt the shea butter, beeswax and olive oil. Once melted, whisk with a hand-held blender for 2 minutes.

2. Add the zinc oxide, borage and the calendula when the mixture has cooled; borage and calendula are fragile oils and their beneficial properties can be destroyed by heat. Continue whisking for 1 minute and leave to stand for 3 minutes.

3. Add the essential oils, then whisk again for a further 2 minutes. Put the whipped balm into a container and label.

ROLL-AWAY BALM

Roll-away balm can be applied to your temples quickly and easily because it is packaged in a roll-on bottle. Because this balm needs to remain fairly liquid, no wax is included.

The essential oil blends are designed for their mood-enhancing properties, so you can use this roll-away balm to calm, energise, soothe, uplift, focus the mind, improve impatience – anything that you can capture in essential oils. This is one of my favourite areas of exploration: how essential oils affect the mind in terms of calming, uplifting, energising and generally influencing the emotions.

Your 'smelling' nerves are your olfactory nerves, which run into the limbic area of your brain, carrying with them odour-identification messages. The brain's limbic area is where perception, memory and discriminative actions are performed. These immediately trigger powerful smell-related emotions and behaviours.

If you feel sad, essential oils can invoke a feeling of happiness, lifting your spirits. If you feel anxious, essential oils can put you at ease and make it easier to deal with a troubling situation. If you feel impatient, essential oils can calm you down, and if you feel a little sluggish, essential oils can put a spring back into your step – all by smell alone. Amazing!

The base ingredients of this roll-away balm are:

5g shea butter
20g avocado oil
10g jojoba oil
20 drops essential oil or blend of essential oils from the list on pages 118–19

Method
1. Melt the shea butter and add it to the avocado and jojoba oils.

2. Add the essential oils and stir well.

3. Put the mixture in roll-on bottles and label them so that you can identify the contents.

Directions for use
Roll a little of the Roll-away Balm onto your temples. Massage your temples until the oil has rubbed into the skin.

Shelf life
• 18 months

Roll-away Balm Mood-enhancing Blends

Wake Up	Cheer Up	Uplifting
5 drops Juniper Berry	8 drops Sweet Orange	8 drops Bergamot
5 drops Lemon	1 drops Grapefruit	3 drops Geranium
5 drops Grapefruit	3 drops Jasmine	3 drops Grapefruit
2 drops Patchouli	6 drops Rose	3 drops Lemon
3 drops Bergamot	2 drops Rosewood	3 drops Lime

Raring to Go	Liberation	Soothe & Calm
2 drops Basil	6 drops Neroli	4 drops Lavender
5 drops Bergamot	2 drops Sweet Orange	2 drops Jasmine
2 drops Grapefruit	2 drops Patchouli	2 drops Myrrh
6 drops Jasmine	6 drops Rose	4 drops Sweet Orange
2 drops Juniper Berry	2 drops Sandalwood	5 drops Rose
3 drops Rosemary	2 drops Ylang-ylang	3 drops Sandalwood

Slow Down, You Move Too Fast	Focus	Energise
2 drops Bay	3 drops Basil	2 drops Basil
2 drops Cedar	4 drops Eucalyptus	4 drops Bergamot
4 drops Chamomile	6 drops Lemon	4 drops Grapefruit
2 drops Eucalyptus	4 drops Peppermint	2 drops Jasmine
4 drops Frankincense	3 drops Rosemary	4 drops Juniper Berry
4 drops Jasmine		4 drops Lemon
2 drops Lavender		

Hangover Fix	Jetlag	Confidence-booster
14 drops Neroli	14 drops Lemon Grass	12 drops Rose
6 drops Sandalwood	3 drops Peppermint	4 drops Geranium
	3 drops Rosemary	2 drops Juniper Berry
		2 drops Lavender

If you prefer to make up your own blends, or to wear just a single oil to help a condition, select the appropriate oil/s from the chart below.

Mood-enhancing essential oils

Tiredness	Depression	Anxiety	Insomnia
Bay	Basil	Basil	Jasmine
Bergamot	Bergamot	Bergamot	Myrrh
Carrot Seed	Chamomile	Carrot Seed	Sweet Orange
Chamomile	Frankincense	Cedar	
Frankincense	Geranium	Chamomile	
Grapefruit	Grapefruit	Frankincense	
Juniper Berry	Jasmine	Geranium	
Lemon	Lavender	Juniper Berry	
Lemon Grass	Lime	Lavender	
Patchouli	Neroli	Lemon Grass	
Peppermint	Sweet Orange	Lime	
Rosemary	Patchouli	Neroli	
Sandalwood	Peppermint	Sweet Orange	
	Rose	Patchouli	
	Rosemary	Rose	
	Rosewood	Sandalwood	
	Sandalwood	Ylang-ylang	
	Ylang-ylang		

Soothing/Calming	Energising	Uplifting	Balancing
Bay	Basil	Bergamot	Geranium
Cedar	Bergamot	Geranium	Lavender
Chamomile	Grapefruit	Grapefruit	Patchouli
Eucalyptus	Jasmine	Lemon	Rose
Frankincense	Juniper Berry	Lime	Rosewood
Jasmine	Lemon	Peppermint	Sandalwood
Lavender	Lemon Grass	Rosemary	
Myrrh	Peppermint	Rosewood	
Neroli	Rosemary	Tea Tree	
Sweet Orange			
Rose			
Rosewood			
Sandalwood			

USING A SERUM

Every skin type needs a burst of additional nourishment from time to time, and this can be addressed easily by using a serum. A serum is an intensive treatment that is highly concentrated yet easily absorbed. Applying a serum under your moisturiser will help the moisturiser better penetrate your skin.

A serum is usually applied to your face after cleansing and toning, but before moisturising because it creates a layer of treatment between the skin and moisturiser. The function of a serum is to boost hydration. This is accomplished by natural moisturising ingredients in the serum and by the fact that it helps moisturiser penetrate your skin quickly and easily. In addition, serum can create a waterproofing layer on your skin, slowing down water loss and thus keeping skin hydrated for longer. A serum works with your moisturiser and should not be relied on as an alternative to moisturising.

Silicones

The main ingredient in commercial serums is a silicone such as cyclomethicone or cyclopentasiloxane, although if you check the ingredients label on the back of your purchased serum container, you may find other silicone ingredients, too.

Silicones and their use in beauty products are a subject of great debate. Personally I think they're fine in moderation – they bring a wonderfully silky feel to skin, they glide smoothly across your face, they're not greasy, they protect skin and they help moisturiser do an even better job since silicone helps it to penetrate better. I would, however, avoid the thicker silicones such as dimethicone, which creates a protective layer but can prevent skin from 'breathing' freely.

Olive squalane

Olive squalane makes an excellent alternative to silicone, although this product is far more costly. Again, it glides across the skin with ease, protects it, feels silky, helps moisturiser to penetrate better and allows skin to breath. Olive squalane is initially a little oilier than non-greasy silicones, but, like the 'on-and-gone' oils, it will sink into your skin, leaving little or no greasy residue.

Olive squalane has the nickname of 'facelift in a bottle' because it has all sorts of wonderful properties that benefit your skin. Squalane is produced naturally by skin until you reach your mid-twenties. Its role is to moisturise and protect.

Olive squalane is similar in molecular structure to human lipids, and is therefore accepted happily and absorbed into skin; it is also suitable for all skin types. Because squalane oil is so fine, it is absorbed deep into skin remarkably quickly. This speedy, deep penetration helps accelerate new cell growth, and because olive squalane also has antibacterial qualities, it can help inhibit the growth of bacteria that can harm normal cell development.

Squalane can be used to soothe and clear rashes and very dry skin patches and will help heal dried and cracked skin on hands, face and other parts of the body. Not surprisingly, this is one of my all-time-favourite versatile ingredients.

While most commercial cosmetic companies build their serums around silicones, in this book, we'll build ours around olive squalane. You can still include silicones with olive squalane if you wish – it helps to bulk out the product, keep costs down and still allows skin to benefit from the wonderful effects brought courtesy of olive squalane.

How & when to use a serum

Unless otherwise instructed, most serums can be applied all over the face. Some are designed to target a particular area, such as around the eyes or wherever skin is prone to fine lines and wrinkles. If a serum has been formulated using a blend of squalane plus other ingredients such as silicone, oils and essential oils, you should shake the serum container before use to ensure all ingredients are mixed together. Put a little of the serum onto the designated areas such as cheekbones, across the area under your nose and above your top lip and gently massage in with clean fingers. Leave to settle for one or two minutes, then apply your moisturiser. Serums can be used once or twice daily.

Serum recipes

Serums are quick and easy to make and require no heating because they're made from liquid ingredients only. Each of the recipes below makes 50g (approximately 50ml) of serum. Since serums are typically packed in a small bottles or tubes that hold anything between 7g–15g, you'll make plenty to last you for a while. A pump bottle is ideal as this will help dispense only a small amount of serum at a time. Serums can also be packaged in bottles that have a dripper or pipette-type dispenser to control the amount of serum dispensed. Because they don't contain water, serums don't require a preservative.

Unless otherwise specified, all serum recipes follow the same method steps and have the same shelf life as the Silky Skin Booster on page 122.

Silky Skin Booster

35g olive squalane
10g cyclomethicone
5g avocado oil

Method
1. Mix the ingredients together and pour into a bottle.

2. Label so that you can identify the contents.

Directions for use
Due to the different weights of the individual liquids, you may find that some separation occurs as the serum is left to stand. Shake the bottle before use to mix the liquids. Place a pea-sized amount of serum on your hands and dot the serum onto cheekbones, chin, nose and forehead. Gently massage the serum into the skin. Apply moisturiser on top of the serum.

Shelf life
• 18 months

Absolute Treat

This is probably the most expensive recipe in the book! However, once you've used the serum and experienced argan oil, you'll probably find yourself justifying the cost quite happily. These two ingredients deserve to have rose essential oil included with them to make this serum an absolute treat.

45g olive squalane
5g argan oil
2 drops rose essential oil

Cell Renewal Serum

Marvellous for dull, tired skin and for mature skin types. Although you can feel the difference straight away, the total benefits of this serum will be most apparent after a few weeks because it takes approximately four to six weeks for new skin cells to become surface skin,

35g olive squalane
10g evening primrose oil
5g avocado oil
4 drops neroli essential oil

Anti-wrinkle Target Serum

Use this serum around the eye area, across the area between top lip and nose and around the jowl line.

35g olive squalane
10g cyclomethicone
5g kukui nut oil
2 drops frankincense essential oil

Eye Serum

Dot this serum around the eye area, including the area between eyelid and eyebrow – being careful not to get any serum in your eye, of course!

46g olive squalane
4g rosehip oil

Lip-prep Serum

This serum is intended to be placed on the lips, preventing chapping and flaking.

40g olive squalane
2g castor oil
1g vitamin E oil
2g jojoba oil

Overnight Secret Serum

Let this serum do its magic while you sleep.

40g olive squalane
5g jojoba oil
5g calendula oil
5 drops jasmine essential oil

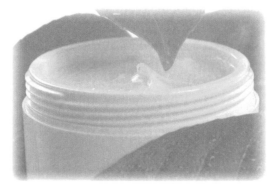

FACIAL OILS

The thought of putting oils directly onto your skin is surprising and not altogether welcomed by many people. If you think all oils are thick, gloopy, greasy and sticky, think again. Such oils would definitely not be contenders as a facial oil – in contrast to thin, light, quickly absorbed, deeply hydrating oils, which are an extremely useful and nourishing skincare beauty treatment.

The right oils offer a wealth of skincare benefits because they contain vitamins, proteins, minerals and other nutrients essential for the development and maintenance of healthy, glowing skin. You can add essential oils to your body oils to give them active, therapeutic qualities as well as making them smell absolutely gorgeous.

Your skin will love facial oils. Contrary to some popular beliefs, putting an oil on your skin will not cause it to be or become greasy, providing you've selected the appropriate type. Your skin produces its own oil, sebum, in an effort to lubricate, protect and moisturise. By using a facial oil you're helping your skin; even an oily skin will soon self-regulate so that it isn't overly greasy.

By understanding the benefits and feel of each oil, you can quickly and easily build a range of blended oils suitable for different uses in skincare. Please see the section on base oils on page 52 for more information on different types of oil properties and behaviour in skincare products.

How & when to use a facial oil

Facial oils can be used as often as you like and whenever you wish. If your skin is very dry, then initially you may need to apply a facial oil two or three times a day, but this does depend on what other skincare treatments you're using.

Facial oils can replace moisturisers, either completely or alternately. For example, you could consider applying a regular moisturiser in the morning and a facial oil at night. You can apply facial oils after using a serum, or you can include oils with olive squalane to make a combination of serum and facial oil.

Facial oil recipes

There are several recipes in this section, starting with the simplest, then moving onto more complex recipes. Any of these oils can double up as body oils. Unless otherwise indicated, all facial oil recipes follow the same method and have the same shelf life as found in the Blessed & Balanced Facial Oil on page 126.

Blessed & Balanced Facial Oil

For mature skins

The oils for this facial oil have been selected for their cell-renewal ability, and for their capacity to firm and improve elasticity, reducing the signs of little lines and wrinkles.

2g vitamin E oil
16g rice bran oil
20g avocado oil
12g evening primrose oil
4 drops neroli essential oil
4 drops frankincense seed oil

Method
1. Place all the ingredients in a small jug or bowl and stir well to combine.

2. Pour the mixture into a bottle and label it so that you can identify the contents.

Directions for use
Place a little of the oil onto each of the cheekbones, forehead, chin and nose and massage into the face in small circles. Leave for 3–4 minutes before applying make-up or additional moisturiser, if required.

Shelf life
• 18–24 months

YOUTHFUL BLOOM SOFT SKIN

50ml jojoba oil
6 drops sandalwood essential oil
6 drops rose essential oil

SKIN-TONING OIL

25ml grapeseed oil
25ml cherry kernel oil
10 drops grapefruit essential oil

PROBLEM SKIN OIL

20ml jojoba oil
20ml avocado oil
7 drops tea tree essential oil
5 drops rosemary essential oil

ANTI-AGING OIL

30ml avocado oil
10ml peach kernel oil
10ml argan oil
8 drops ylang-ylang essential oil
4 drops frankincense essential oil

Hydrating & Healing

20ml avocado oil
20ml jojoba oil
10ml argan oil
6 drops lavender essential oil
3 drops rosewood essential oil
2 drops elemi essential oil

Help Me Hydrate Oil

25ml avocado oil
25ml jojoba oil
6 drops sweet orange essential oil
6 drops cedar essential oil

Purity Facial Oil

For problem skin

The oils chosen for this facial oil have been selected for their antibacterial, anti-inflammatory, healing and soothing qualities.

2g vitamin E oil
20g flaxseed oil
15g jojoba oil
13g rosehip oil
2 drops bergamot essential oil
2 drops chamomile oil
3 drops juniper berry essential oil

ANTIOXIDANT FACIAL OIL

For combination skin

This oil will actually suit most skin types, but it is especially suitable for combination skins, due to the rebalancing elements of the jojoba and geranium and lavender essential oils.

5g vitamin E oil
30g jojoba oil
15g sweet almond oil
3 drops lavender essential oil
3 drops geranium essential oil
2 drops rosemary essential oil

REJUVENATING FACIAL OIL

For dry skin

Rejuvenating Facial Oil will help hydrate dry skin while providing soothing, anti-itch and anti-inflammatory capabilities, courtesy of the apricot kernel, calendula and flaxseed oils. The rose and chamomile essential oils further boost the hydration and will leave your skin feeling soft and supple.

1g vitamin E oil
20g apricot kernel oil
20g flaxseed oil
9g calendula oil
4 drops rose essential oil
4 drops chamomile essential oil

Soothing Facial Oil
For sensitive skin

This facial oil is suitable for the most sensitive of skin types and has been formulated with soothing, nourishing and protective oils of macadamia nut, melon seed and safflower. The essential oils of rosewood and sandalwood are soothing and comforting.

1g vitamin E oil
30g melon seed oil
10g safflower oil
9g macadamia nut oil
3 drops rosewood essential oil
3 drops sandalwood oil

Regulating Facial Oil
For oily skin

Facial oils suitable for oily skin help regulate sebum and encourage the sebaceous glands to re-cue their natural oil production. Grapeseed oil will refine and close pores while the essential oils of clary sage, geranium and grapefruit will help decongest blocked pores and also limit overproduction of sebum.

1g vitamin E oil
20g grapeseed oil
20g jojoba oil
9g hazelnut oil
3 drops clary sage essential oil
2 drops geranium essential oil
2 drops grapefruit essential oil

PICK-UP HEALING FACIAL OIL
For tired, dull skin

This oil is wonderful when you're feeling a little sluggish and worn out. It's an instant pick-me-up in terms of aroma-utilising essential oils that will perk up dull, lifeless skin. The base oils include rosehip, grapeseed and blackcurrant seed oils for their immune-boosting, rejuvenating, healing and nourishing abilities.

1g vitamin E oil
5g rosehip oil
10g grapeseed oil
34g blackcurrant seed oil
4 drops sweet orange essential oil
2 drops juniper berry essential oil
2 drops bergamot essential oil

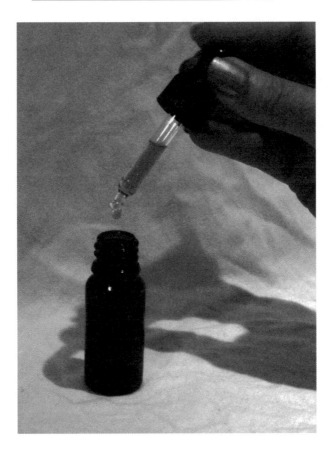

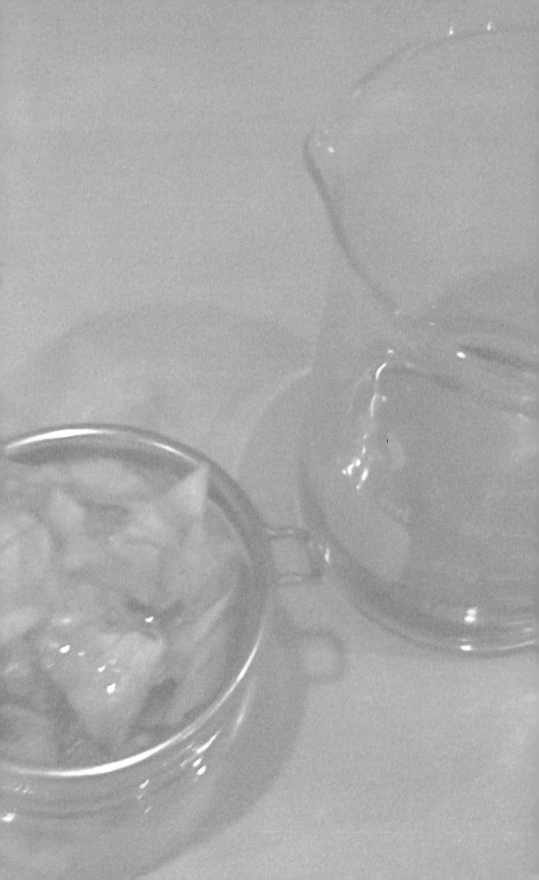

CHAPTER 7

Making Tinctures & Infusions

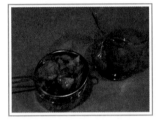

As you have seen by now, plant materials contain properties that are helpful to your skin. Just as in the case of base oils and essential oils, it is possible to extract these beneficial properties into oils, water and alcohol, then use these plant liquids when creating your own skincare products. They may not be as concentrated as essential oils, but they will still contribute useful properties.

In this chapter you'll discover how to make oil infusions, water infusions, decoctions and tinctures – none of which are difficult to do, and each one will contribute slightly different properties to the care of your skin. Being able to make an infusion, for instance, opens up a whole new world when it comes to creating skincare products. Any herb, flower or plant material can be used, provided you've carried out sufficient research to ensure that the plant is safe to use on your skin.

While it is possible to collect herbs and flowers from your garden, hedgerows and other permitted outdoor areas, do make sure that you wash the plant material and leave it to dry naturally. Purchasing dried herbs and flowers from reputable sources is a safer way of ensuring that the plant material is clean and pesticide-free.

The chart on pages 140–1 provides a list of common plants that are suitable for making infusions, decoctions and tinctures, as well as their beneficial qualities and suitability for various skin types.

INFUSED OILS

Infused oils are similar to essential oils in that they contain beneficial properties from the plants from which they are extracted. Unlike essential oils, however, infused herbal oils are not volatile; they don't evaporate and therefore have little or no smell. This can make them the perfect ingredient for skincare products where the aroma of an essential oil may be overpowering or unwanted. Infused oils are not as concentrated as essential oils and can be used directly on skin without having to dilute them further. Making a herbal infusion can be done easily at home because it doesn't require any special equipment other than the bowls and jars you probably already have in your cupboards.

How to make an oil infusion

To make a herbal infusion, you will need a clean jar with a tightly fitting lid, a supply of herbs (or petals or other plant material) and a base oil. The base oil will absorb the properties of the herbs when left to steep for a number of days. Suitable base oils include sunflower, olive and sweet almond oil.

Herbal oil infusion: cold method (also known as the sun method)

1. Chop your dried herbs or petals into fine pieces to smooth the progress of the infusion of the plant's properties into the oil.

2. Put the chopped herbs or flowers into a clean jar. Fill the jar as much as you can. Cover the herbs or flowers completely with your chosen oil and fill the jar to the rim with oil. Make sure all the plant pieces are completely submerged in the oil.

3. Replace the lid and label the jar so that you can identify its contents. Include the date you started the infusion as part of the label information.

4. Place the jar on a sunny window sill or in the sunshine somewhere and leave to steep for at least 10 days. If the sunlight is very strong, move the jar to a cooler (but still sunny) spot.

5. Shake the jar vigorously every day.

6. After 10 days, strain the oil through a strainer, straining bag or piece of muslin to separate the herbs from the oil. Pour the infused oil in a clean jar, preferably one made of dark glass. Label the jar so that you can identify the contents.

Directions for use
This oil can be used to replace any of the base oils in any of the recipes in this book. For a more intense, concentrated oil, repeat the process with a fresh batch of chopped herbs or petals, but infuse them in the same oil that you've already used to make the first infusion. The same oil can be used for two or three sessions, using a new batch of chopped plant material each time.

The characteristic of the oil will be taken from the type of base oil you used. If you infused in sunflower oil, for example, then the oil will have a medium absorption speed and medium absorption ability. If you infused your herbs in avocado oil, then the infused oil will be an on-and-gone oil: quick to absorb, with thorough absorption capabilities. What makes the infused oil different is that it now has the benefits and qualities you extracted from the plant.

Shelf life
• 12 months

Herbal infusion: hot method
This method is quicker because it uses a heat source to encourage the herbs to release their properties into the oil. It is not suitable for fragile base oils, however, because the heat can destroy some of the properties of the oil itself.

1. Chop the plant material into small pieces and put them in a clean, heatproof bowl.

2. Cover the herbs with your chosen oil and stand the bowl in a pan of simmering water. Gently heat the herbs and oil and leave to steep for 1 hour. Turn off the heat and let the oil cool, then turn the heat on and bring the pan water up to simmering again. Do not allow the oil to get too hot; you don't want it to start cooking.

3. Remove the infused oil from the heat and strain through a sieve, straining bag or muslin cloth to remove any trace of plant material. Allow the mixture to cool before bottling. Label the container so that you can identify the contents.

As an alternative to the bowl-over-simmering-water method, put the chopped herbs and oil in a slow cooker and leave it on slow heat for 4 hours. You can re-infuse hot-method oils several times with a new set of fresh or dried herbs to make double- or triple-strength infused oils.

Shelf life
• 12 months

INFUSED WATERS

Making an infused water is even easier than making an oil infusion – the process is as simple as making a pot of tea. No surprise, then, that a water infusion is also known as a tea, a tisane or a rinse.

Fresh and dried flower petals and herbs make excellent plant material for a water infusion. While infused waters can be used to replace or blend with floral water and spring water in any of the recipes in this book, please note that a preservative must be used in order to keep the product fresh for more than a couple of days. Otherwise, keep your infused waters in the fridge and use them within one week of making them.

How to make a water infusion

1. Chop your dried herbs or petals into fine pieces. Put these into a heatproof jug or bowl.

2. Pour boiling water over the plant pieces and leave it to steep for 10 minutes. Strain through a piece of muslin or a fine strainer.

Directions for use
Use instead of water or floral water in any of the recipes in this book.

Shelf life for any product made with a water infusion
• 1 week without preservative, kept in the refrigerator
• 4 months, with preservative

DECOCTIONS

A decoction is made by boiling the woodier, denser, more fibrous parts of a plant such as its roots, berries, seeds and bark.

How to make a decoction

1. Roughly chop up the plant material into smaller chunks and put them in a large stainless-steel saucepan with a close-fitting lid.

2. Pour over enough water to immerse the chopped plant pieces completely, making sure they're all below the water line.

3. Slowly bring the pan to the boil. Allow the water to simmer for 15 minutes, then strain through a muslin cloth or strainer.

4. Store in a lidded container and label it so that you can identify the contents.

Directions for use
Use the decoction to replace all or some of the spring water or floral waters in any of the recipes in this book.

Shelf life for any product made with a decoction
• 1 week without preservative, kept in the refrigerator
• 4 months, with preservative

TINCTURES

Tinctures are a mixture of alcohol and plant material; the process used in making a tincture is called maceration. In this case, the plant material can be taken from any part of the plant, such as petals, whole flower heads and stalks, herb leaves, berries, pods, bark and roots. Tinctures are also known as extracts – although, confusingly, extracts are also the name given to plant material that has been extracted into other liquids, such as glycerine and propylyl glycol.

When making a tincture, it is the alcohol, glycerine or propylyl glycol that extracts the beneficial properties from the plant and captures them in the liquid. Suitable alcohols to use are ethyl alcohol, isopropyl (rubbing) alcohol, denatured alcohol or vodka. This alcohol should never be consumed, however; even if vodka is used as the extracting agent, remember that in this case it is *for topical skincare products only.*

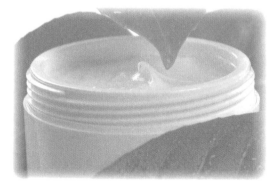

How to make a tincture

1. Take 3–4 handfuls of your chosen plant material (or combination of plant materials) and grind or chop it into small pieces – the smaller the pieces, the better the tincture.

2. Put the crushed plant material into a glass jar and fill it with alcohol so that the plant material is submerged. Ideally fill the jar with the plant material, then fill up to the neck of the jar with your chosen alcohol, ensuring that no part of the plant material is exposed to air. Put the lid on the jar and give the mixture a shake.

3. Put the jar in a cool cupboard for at least 2 weeks. Shake it daily to mix the plant material with the alcohol.

4. At the end of the 2-week period (or longer), strain the liquid through a piece of muslin, fine-mesh sieve or filter paper (the filter papers used for coffee machines make useful tincture filter papers).

5. Pour the liquid into a dark glass bottle. Be sure to label it so that you can identify the contents.

Directions for use
You only require a little tincture in skincare products – usually between 3–10%. The tinctures are an addition to the ingredients used in the recipes in this book and they can make a particularly beneficial supplement to cleansers and face masks, although they aren't limited to these products.

Tinctures should not be applied directly to the face, however, because the alcohol content may make them unnecessarily drying.

Shelf life
• 12 months

Plant types and skin suitability

Plant	Part used	Benefits	Suitable for skin types
Borage	Leaves and petals	Soothes damaged and irritated skin, reduces reddening, regenerative	Oily, sensitive, mature, dry
Calendula (Marigold)	Petals	Calming, soothing, healing, anti-inflammatory	Dry
Carrot	Vegetable root	Restorative for dry, damaged skin	Dry, sensitive, mature
Chamomile	Petals	Soothing, anti-irritant, calming	Dry, sensitive
Elderflower	Petals	Mildly astringent, anti-inflammatory, boosts immune system, healing	Oily, combination, sensitive
Green Tea	Leaves	Antioxidant, anti-inflammatory, improves skin's elasticity	All skin types
- Hibiscus	Petals and stalk	Antioxidant, healing, restorative for dry, damaged skin, astringent	Dry, combination
Juniper	Berries and stems	Anti-inflammatory, decongests blocked pores	Dry
Lavender	Flower head	Soothing, healing, anti-itch	Combination
Lemon Balm	Leaves	Antibacterial, cleansing	Oily
Marshmallow	Leaves and root	Antibacterial, anti-inflammatory, healing	Dry, sensitive
Milk Thistle	All	Antioxidant	Oily
Nettle	Leaves	Anti-inflammatory, antioxidant, soothing	Mature, combination

Plant types and skin suitability

Plant	Part used	Benefits	Suitable for skin types
Patchouli	Leaves	Encourages skin cell regeneration, healing, anti-inflammatory, fights infections	All
Peppermint	Leaves	Cooling, soothing, anti-itch, reduces redness	All
Rose	Petals	Anti-inflammatory, reduces redness, hydrating	Dry, combination, sensitive, mature
Rosehip	Fruit	Healing, rejuvenating, anti-aging	Dry, sensitive. mature
Rosemary	Leaves and stalk	Antioxidant, stimulating, antibacterial	Oily
Sage	Leaves	Regulates sebum, healing, antibacterial, anti-inflammatory, antiseptic, astringent	Combination, oily
St John's Wort	Leaves	Cooling, astringent, calming, anti-inflammatory	Sensitive, dry
Witch Hazel	Leaves, twigs, bark	Astringent, anti-inflammatory	Oily

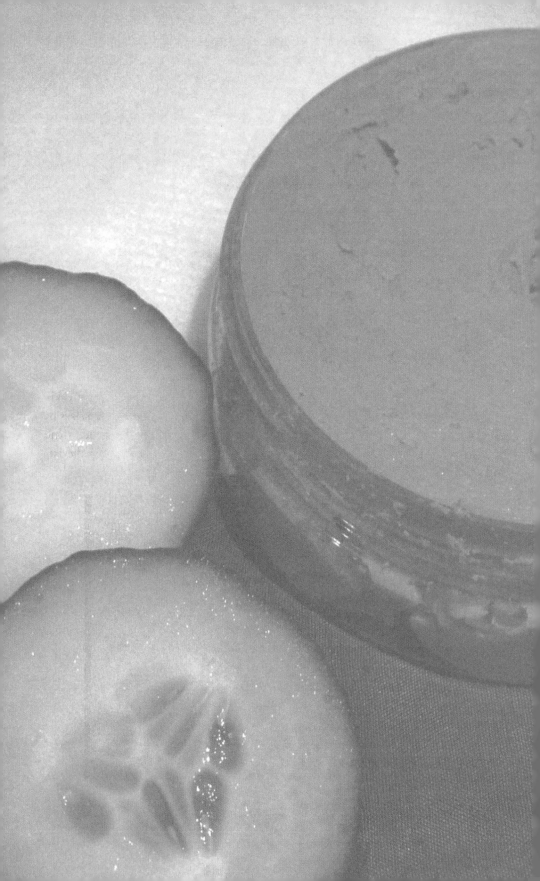

CHAPTER 8

Treatments for Troubled Skin: Rosacea, Acne & Eczema

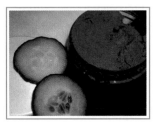

Although these skin conditions are never welcome, there are times when your skin is more prone to various symptoms of these complaints. We can help ourselves by having a healthy lifestyle, balanced diet and a regular exercise routine – and thankfully, a variety of natural active ingredients have been proven to help alleviate these problems, too.

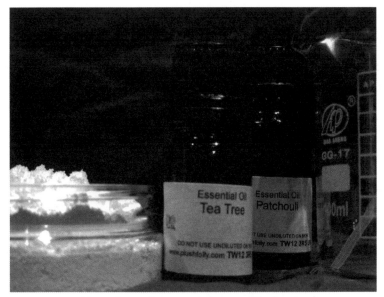

Natural ingredients can help treat skin disorders

ROSACEA

Rosacea is a common inflammatory skin condition that is characterised by redness to the face, which looks like a deep blush. It comes and goes and is often triggered by hot drinks, alcohol and spicy foods.

Rosacea is sometimes called acne rosacea, which is misleading because rosacea and acne are two totally different conditions (although they can occur together). There is no complete cure for rosacea, but because this condition comes and goes, some of the following natural ingredients may help to reduce its occurrence – and offer relief when it does occur. Signs of rosacea include:

- Red patches on the face and flushed cheeks,
- Small red bumps or raised blotches on cheeks, forehead and nose

Base oils to help treat rosacea include:

- Evening primrose oil,
- Flaxseed oil, and
- Borage oil.

Use these oils in your moisturising or night creams, or make a facial oil using the oils on their own or in a blend.

Herbal treatments for rosacea include:

- Chrysanthellum indicum extract,
- Green tea,
- Chamomile, and
- Burdock.

Use the herbs and flowers to make an oil or water infusion and apply the infusion to the affected area, either directly or in a cream or other carrier product such as a gentle non-drying mask or gel.

Essential oils to help treat rosacea include:

- Lavender,
- Chamomile,
- Tea tree, and
- Rose.

Replace the essential oils in any of the moisturising or night cream recipes with lavender, chamomile, tea tree or rose, or a combination of these oils.

Other natural ingredients to help treat rosacea include:

- Oatmeal,
- Aloe vera, and
- Zinc oxide.

Apply the ingredients to the affected areas in a skincare treatment such as a gentle non-drying mask or gel.

Rosacea treatment recipes

Using the ingredients that can help treat rosacea and the recipes listed earlier in this book, you can formulate your own rosacea remedies. I have included a few to get you started.

ROSACEA FACIAL OIL TREATMENT

25g evening primrose oil
10g flaxseed oil
10g borage oil
5g vitamin E oil
6 drops lavender essential oil
4 drops tea tree essential oil

1. Mix all the ingredients together. Put the mixture into a suitable labelled container.

2. Apply twice daily directly to the face using a cotton-wool pad or clean fingers.

Shelf life
- 12 months

Rosacea Soothing Night Cream

15g flaxseed oil
5g beeswax
8g emulsifying wax NF
50g rose water
5g vitamin E oil
15g borage oil
4 drops rose essential oil
2 drops chamomile essential oil
0.5g preservative (optional)

1. Put the flaxseed, beeswax and emulsifying wax in a heatproof jug or bowl and stand the bowl in a pan of simmering water. Stir to encourage the waxes to melt.

2. Put the rose water and preservative (if using) in another heatproof jug or bowl and stand this in a pan of simmering water.

3. Once the waxes have melted and the rose water has warmed through, combine the ingredients and stir well. Add the vitamin E and borage oil and continue to stir until the mixture starts to cool and thicken. Add the essential oils, preservative if using and stir again. Once the mixture has cooled, put the cream in a suitable labelled container.

4. Apply directly to a clean face twice daily.

Shelf life
• 4 weeks without preservative
• 9 months with preservative

Rosacea Gentle Facial Mask

10g cooled chamomile water infusion
(see Making Tinctures and Infusions, page 136)
10g aloe vera
0.5g xanthan gum
10g pink clay
5g white clay
3g zinc oxide
3g evening primrose oil
3 drops chamomile essential oil

1. Put the chamomile water and aloe vera in a small bowl and sprinkle over the xanthan gum, clays and zinc oxide. Leave for 1 minute, then stir the powders into the water. Add the evening primrose oil and chamomile essential oil and stir again.

2. Adjust the water or clay to achieve the correct consistency, then put the mask into a suitable labelled container. Keep it in the refrigerator.

3. Apply a thin layer onto your face, avoiding the eye and lip areas. Leave the mask on for 15 minutes, then wash off with tepid water. Apply a generous helping of moisturiser after using the mask.

Shelf life
Because this mask doesn't contain a preservative, keep for a maximum of 2 weeks in the refrigerator.

ACNE

Acne is quite a common skin condition and is often suffered by teenagers experiencing hormonal changes. Acne spots appear as blackheads, whiteheads and small pink bumps. The cause of acne is usually blocked oil glands, which trap sebum, causing inflammation and infection.

Acne can be cured, but often the sufferer is left with scarring. Once the acne has cleared up, use vitamin E or rosehip oil either directly or in a skincare treatment to help reduce the scarring.

Signs of acne include:

- Red bumps on the face, shoulders, back and other parts of the body,
- Red bumps with a yellow head, and
- Blackheads on red, inflamed skin.

A key factor in keeping acne at bay is to have a clean, oil-free face. Make sure you cleanse regularly and remove all traces of make-up and cleanser before going to bed. Base oils to help treat acne include:

- Castor oil,
- Jojoba oil,
- Coconut oil, and
- Rosehip oil.

Use these oils in your moisturising or night creams or make a facial oil using these oils on their own or in a blend.

Herbal treatments for acne include:

- Green tea,
- Red clover,
- Burdock,
- Dandelion, and
- Nettles.

Use the herbs to make an oil or water infusion and apply the infusion to the affected area, either directly, in a light moisturising cream or in another carrier product such as a clay mask or gel.

Essential oils to help treat acne include:

- Tea tree,
- Bergamot,
- Clary sage,
- Eucalyptus,
- Geranium,
- Lavender, and
- Roman chamomile.

Use a few drops of the essential oil in a skincare treatment such as a clay mask or gel.

Other natural ingredients to help treat acne include:

- Aloe vera,
- Witch hazel,
- Zinc oxide, and
- Fuller's earth.

Apply the ingredients to the affected areas in a skincare treatment such as a gentle non-drying mask or gel.

Acne treatment recipes

Using the ingredients that can help treat acne and the recipes listed earlier in this book, you can formulate your own acne remedies. Here are a few to get you started.

ACNE FACIAL OIL TREATMENT

25g jojoba oil
10g fractionated coconut oil
10g rosehip oil
5g castor oil
8 drops tea tree essential oil
2 drops bergamot essential oil

1. Mix all the ingredients together and put in a suitable labelled container.

2. Apply twice daily directly to the face using a cotton-wool pad or clean fingers.

Shelf life
- 12 months

ACNE SOOTHING NIGHT CREAM

20g jojoba oil
5g rosehip oil
5g coconut oil
10g emulsifying wax NF
20g tea tree water
30g witch hazel
0.5g preservative (optional)
4 drops tea tree essential oil
2 drops lavender essential oil

1. Put the jojoba, rosehip and coconut oils and emulsifying wax in a heatproof jug or bowl and stand the bowl in a pan of simmering water. Stir to encourage the wax to melt.

2. Put the tea tree water, witch hazel and preservative (if using) in another heatproof jug or bowl and stand this in a pan of simmering water.

3. Once the waxes have melted and the tea tree water and witch hazel have warmed through, combine the ingredients and stir well. When the mixture begins to cool and thicken, add the essential oils and stir again.

4. Once the mixture has cooled, put the cream in a suitable labelled container.

5. Apply directly to a clean face twice daily.

Shelf life
• 4 weeks without preservative
• 9 months with preservative

ACNE DEEP-TREATMENT FACIAL MASK

10g cooled nettle water infusion (see Making Tinctures & Infusions, page 136)
10g aloe vera
0.5g preservative (optional)
10g fuller's earth
5g Dead Sea mud
3g zinc oxide
3g jojoba oil
3 drops bergamot essential oil

1. Put the nettle water, aloe vera and preservative (if using) in a small bowl and sprinkle over the fuller's earth, Dead Sea mud and zinc oxide. Leave for 1 minute, then stir the powders into the water.

2. Add the jojoba oil and bergamot essential oil and stir again.

3. Adjust the water or clay to achieve the correct consistency, then put the mask into a suitable labelled container.

4. Apply a thin layer onto your face, avoiding the eye and lip areas. Leave the mask on for 15 minutes, then wash off with tepid water. Apply a generous helping of moisturiser after using the mask.

Shelf life
• 2 weeks without preservative, kept in the refrigerator
• 3 months with preservative

ECZEMA

Eczema is a skin disorder in which the skin becomes overly dry, itchy and inflamed. It can be cured, but often the cause isn't known. It's not uncommon for treated eczema to disappear, yet return again without any apparent reason. Signs of eczema include:

- Dry, flaky patches,
- Red inflamed and swollen patches,
- Cracked skin, and
- Blistered, weeping skin.

Base oils and butters to help treat eczema include:

- Calendula oil,
- Neem oil,
- Vitamin E oil,
- Borage oil,
- Cocoa butter,
- Shea butter, and
- Oils rich in gamma-linolenic acid (GLA).

Apply the oils directly to your face or in a skincare treatment such as a moisturising cream, balm, gel or face oil.

Herbal treatments for eczema include:

- Comfrey,
- Nettles, and
- Calendula.

Use the herbs to make an oil or water infusion and apply the infusion to the affected area either directly or in a light cream.

Essential oils to help eczema include:

- Bergamot (weepy eczema),
- Juniper (weepy eczema),
- Clary sage (dry eczema),
- Lavender (dry eczema),
- Geranium (dry eczema), and
- Roman chamomile (dry eczema).

Use a few drops of the essential oil in a skincare treatment such as a cream or balm.

Other natural ingredients to help eczema include:

- Oatmeal, and
- Zinc oxide.

Apply the ingredients to the affected areas in a skincare treatment such as a gentle non-drying mask or gel.

To make an oatmeal bath: add a handful of oatmeal to a warm (not hot) bath and immerse yourself for five minutes. Gently pat yourself dry with a towel and apply moisturiser while the skin is still damp.

A blend of honey, olive oil and melted beeswax used as a treatment and left on the skin for 20 minutes can be beneficial and soothing for inflamed, dry eczema patches.

Eczema treatment recipes

Using the ingredients that can help treat eczema and the recipes listed earlier in this book, you can formulate your own eczema remedies. Here are a few to get you started.

ECZEMA FACIAL OIL TREATMENT

25g calendula oil
15g melon seed oil
10g rosehip oil
5g vitamin E oil
4 drops chamomile essential oil
2 drops rose essential oil

1. Mix all the ingredients together and put in suitable labelled container.

2. Apply twice daily directly to the face using a cotton-wool pad or clean fingers.

Shelf life
- 12 months

ECZEMA SOOTHING NIGHT CREAM

15g calendula oil
15g shea butter
5g beeswax
8g emulsifying wax NF
50g rose geranium (or geranium) water
0.5g preservative (optional)
5g vitamin E oil
4 drops geranium essential oil
2 drops chamomile essential oil

1. Put the calendula oil, shea butter, beeswax and emulsifying wax in a heatproof jug or bowl and stand the bowl in a pan of simmering water. Stir to encourage the waxes to melt.

2. Put the rose geranium water and preservative (if using) in another heatproof jug or bowl and stand this in a pan of simmering water.

3. Once the waxes have melted and the rose geranium water has warmed through, combine the two and stir well. Add the vitamin E and continue to stir until the mixture starts to cool and thicken.

4. Add the essential oils and stir again. Once the mixture has cooled, put the cream into a suitable labelled container.

5. Apply directly to a clean face twice daily.

Shelf life
• 4 weeks with preservative
• 9 months without preservative

Eczema Gentle Facial Mask

5g oats
10g cooled nettle water infusion
(see Making Tinctures and Infusions, page 136)
35g spring water
0.5g preservative (optional)
0.5g xanthan gum
5g pink clay
3g calendula oil
3 drops lavender essential oil

---

1. Put the oats in a pestle and mortar and crush them to a fine powder.

2. Put the nettle and spring waters and preservative (if using) in a bowl and sprinkle over the xanthan gum, crushed oat powder and clay. Leave to stand for 1 minute, then stir the powders into the waters.

3. Add the calendula oil and lavender essential oil and stir again.

4. Add more water if the mixture is too thick, then put the mask treatment into a suitable labelled container.

5. Apply a thin layer onto your face, avoiding the eye and lip areas. Leave the mask on for 15 minutes, then wash off with tepid water. Apply a generous helping of moisturiser after using the mask.

Shelf life
• 2 weeks without preservative, kept in the refrigerator
• 3 months with preservative

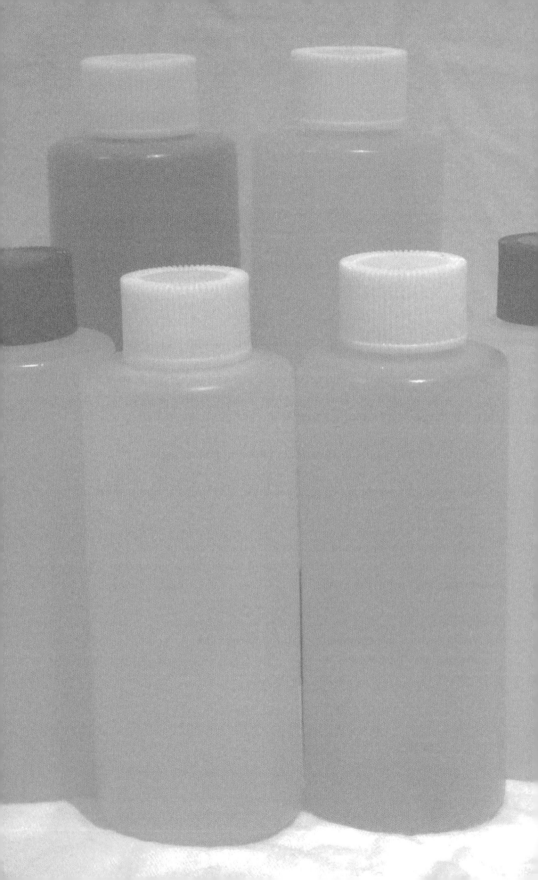

CHAPTER 9

Emulsions, Antioxidants & Preservatives

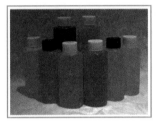

Every individual ingredient included in your skincare product plays an important role. Three of the most important ingredients to consider when making skincare preparations are emulsifiers, antioxidants and preservatives.

Emulsifiers are used to combine ingredients that don't naturally mix, such as water and oils. They are used extensively in all types of creams and lotions and usually take the form of a wax or a liquid, depending on the texture and consistency of the final product. If you're making a cream or lotion, an emulsifier is a compulsory ingredient.

An antioxidant is an optional, extremely beneficial ingredient which can be included in almost all skincare products. Antioxidants have two key functions: to slow down the damage caused to skin by exposure to sun and the environment, and also to help prevent delicate oils from deteriorating quickly once they are exposed to the air. Many natural ingredients contain a rich source of antioxidants, and these can easily be included in skincare products to reduce the sign of sun damage and therefore slow down the signs of ageing.

Preservatives are used to prevent the growth of bacteria and other unwanted, potentially dangerous microbes. Skincare products that don't contain water, such as balms or salves, don't necessarily require a preservative, but if you include water in your preparations, you should consider adding one. There are many different types of preservative, some more natural than others, some easier to use than others, and some more cost effective than others. All serve the same purpose, which is to keep skincare products free from unwanted bacteria, fungus, yeast and mould.

WATER & OIL EMULSIONS

Water and oil emulsions are used extensively in the world of cosmetics (and beyond – think mayonnaise or paint). A face cream, body lotion, hand cream, hair conditioner and creamy cleansers are all forms of water and oil emulsions. Water and oil don't mix together naturally and need the helping hand of an extra ingredient: an emulsifier.

Emulsifying ingredients

An emulsifying ingredient has the task of combining two immiscible liquids. Immiscible means 'not compatible', and therefore not able to mix together to make a solution. Oil and water (for skincare products), or oil and vinegar (for culinary products), are perfect examples of two immiscible liquids.

Water-loving materials are hydrophilic (*hydro* meaning water, *philic* meaning 'loving' or 'friend'), while water-hating materials are hydrophobic (*phobic* meaning fear). Oils are hydrophobic and don't want to mix with water. However, in order to bind water and oil, the two ingredients need to be attracted to each other with a view to staying together.

To overcome this incompatibility and combine them, we need to add two vital ingredients: energy and an emulsifying agent. Emulsifying agents have both a hydrophilic and a hydrophobic element, which allow them to act as a 'dating agency'. This means that the emulsifier is attractive to both oil and water and allows them to unite and remain locked together in an embrace. In the case of skincare products, the energy comes in the form of agitation, either by hand-stirring or whisking, or in the form of mechanical whisking, beating, etc.

The emulsifier is the ingredient that allows the water and oil to bind together to form a moisturising skincare cream or lotion. But we don't just limit emulsifiers to skincare; emulsifiers are used in many food preparations as well. Imagine a salad dressing made with oil and vinegar. Although you can shake and whisk the two ingredients together, when left to stand, the oil and vinegar gradually separate to return to two distinct liquids. Over any given period of time, even an emulsified product may become unstable and separate back into its original form.

When the same ingredients, oil and vinegar, are used in mayonnaise, however, this time they are energized, usually by an electric blender, and emulsified with an egg yolk. The egg yolk will bind and hold the ingredients so that they don't separate, but combine into a rich, creamy product instead.

While you could potentially use an egg yolk to help emulsify your skincare oil and water products, the shelf life would be extremely short. Instead, you need to use an emulsifier that is suitable for use in skincare products and therefore suitable for use on skin.

Emulsifiers don't just combine immiscible liquids; they also work hard to ensure that once the ingredients have been bound together, they remain together without separating. In skincare terms this is known as stabilising products. So the function of an emulsifier becomes twofold: the first function is to combine and the second function is to stabilise the two liquids.

In addition, emulsifiers are formulated so that they bring other properties and abilities to your products, such as a silky skin feel, a good glide across the skin upon application or the ability to thicken the final product.

Emulsifying wax

Emulsifying wax, also known as e-wax, started out life as a natural product. Emulsifying waxes are derived from coconut, palm, olive and other vegetable oils, but their natural composition has been modified to create a product with a function. In the case of an emulsifying wax this is a vegetable-derived wax that has been modified to ensure it is a reliable emulsifier and thickening agent and the chances of the oil and waters separating are very low.

Many different types of emulsifying waxes are available and I recommend that you experiment to find one that works best for your combinations of oils, waters and other included ingredients – and that fits within your budget.

A reliable emulsifier is emulsifying wax NF. The NF or 'National Formulary' means that it is accepted for use in products worldwide. On a skincare product label it will be listed as cetearyl alcohol (and) polysorbate 60.

Emulsifying waxes, which are usually sold under their brand names, are a combination of similar ingredients. More often than not they have been incorporated with cetearyl alcohol, a fatty alcohol made from natural oils and fats (cetyl and stearyl alcohol), which acts as a stabiliser and thickener. On its own, cetearyl alcohol will not bind oils and waters, but it will help prevent the mixture from separating in its container.

Some emulsifying waxes are formulated with cetearyl alcohol combined with PEG-20 stearate, a synthetic compound from the PEG group. PEG stands for polyethylene glycol, which is used in cosmetic products to help active ingredients better penetrate the skin. Different PEGs have different functions. In the case of our emulsifying wax, the PEG-20 stearate is used to combine and hold oil and water, thus performing a vital function in emulsifying wax.

Other emulsifying waxes include emulsifying wax BP (British Pharmacopeia), olivem, BTMS (behentrimonium methosulfate and cetearyl alcohol) and cetearyl glucoside, although this is only a small selection of what's available. They all perform exactly the same function but have slightly different properties when it comes to thickening a product, its texture on the skin, etc.

Lecithin

You may recognise this ingredient. It is commonly used in foods, especially chocolate. If you think about milk chocolate, you have a combination of cocoa bean mass, cocoa butter, milk and sugar (and other ingredients) bound into a solid. This mixture needs emulsifying; because cocoa butter is a fat and milk is a liquid, the two ingredients don't want to mix together – just like the oil and water in face creams.

So chocolatiers have the issue of the cocoa butter and the milk being immiscible, but thankfully lecithin comes to the rescue as an emulsifier and binds and holds the chocolate ingredients together. Lecithin is obtained from soya and also from egg, which is why eggs are used to make mayonnaise. Lecithin is thick and gloopy and looks a little like treacle. Every time I use it, I find myself licking my lips!

Lecithin can also be used to emulsify skincare creams. Since it is such a dark, heavy, treacle-like substance, it can be difficult to measure accurately because it either wants to stick to dispensing equipment or dollop out in far bigger quantities than are needed. The dark colour will definitely have an impact on the final colour of your cream, making it pale golden rather than the usual white.

Lecithin also has water-retention abilities and will help keep your skin moisturised over a longer period of time. I often use a combination of lecithin and emulsifying wax when formulating a cream.

Liquid emulsifiers

If you have an oil and water combination you wish to keep as a liquid, wax is not an appropriate choice as an emulsifier. Cleansing waters, room sprays (which have essential oils as the oil component) and bath oils (where the bath oil needs to disperse into the bath water) are examples of desirable oil and water combinations, or liquid emulsions.

Liquid emulsifiers include polysorbate 20, polysorbate 80, sucragel and sulphonated castor oil. Polysorbates are derived from vegetable oils. Polysorbate 20 is coconut-oil-based and polysorbate 80 is olive-oil-based. Polysorbate 20 is lighter than polysorbate 80 and more suitable for room and linen sprays, whereas polysorbate 80 is an ideal ingredient for bath oils.

Sucragel is derived from sugars – in the form of either sweet almond oil or coconut oil, depending on the variety – while sulphonated castor oil is derived from castor oil. It is also known as turkey red oil – even though it is neither red nor has anything to do with turkeys!

As with any functional ingredient, have fun experimenting until you find the most appropriate emulsifier for your partcular blend of ingredients. Although the general rule of thumb is to make 5–15% of your total product the emulsifying ingredient, you should experiment with different quantities to observe what impact they have on your final skincare product.

Borax

Many skincare books refer to a borax and beeswax combination as being a reliable natural emulsifying agent to use in creams and lotions. It should be noted that borax is a potential skin irritant and as such, my recommendation is to avoid using it in any form of skincare product.

Within the EU, borax is a restricted ingredient in skincare and bath products. Therefore no matter how well it performs, I don't advise that you start formulating with borax. It does, however, still appear in many commercially manufactured cosmetic products as 'sodium borate'.

If you do wish to use borax, then use it only in very small amounts and patch test your product before use. To use borax in a cream, dissolve it in the floral or spring waters while they're being heated.

You can purchase borax in larger supermarkets. Tesco has started selling big boxes of it as part of its 'natural laundry' range.

Beeswax

The humble honeybee didn't design beeswax to be an emulsifier, yet on those occasions where it successfully binds and holds oils and waters, it makes a delightful and very rich cream. As with all bee products (beeswax, propolis and honey), the therapeutic benefits are well known for helping very dry, itchy skin as well as for their antibacterial qualities.

Using beeswax as an emulsifier can produce varying degrees of success. When used with borax, the results are stable – but we have discussed borax above and possibly dismissed it as an unsuitable ingredient. This is a shame, because beeswax and borax make a fabulous partnership and for those who aren't sensitive to borax, beautiful creams can be created by using these two ingredients to emulsify.

If you do decide to use beeswax to emulsify your water and oils, then use it in exactly the same way as you would emulsifying wax NF in any of the recipes in this book. Once the waters, melted beeswax and oils have been combined, stir continuously as the cream cools. If you find the cream attempting to curdle and split, put it back on a low heat and continue to stir until the mixture re-forms and holds together. Remove it from the heat and stir until cool.

If the mixture splits and you give up trying to bring it back together, don't despair! Tip out the water seeping from the cream; you will eventually end up with a very thick dollop of cream. While this might not look fluffy, creamy and attractive, it makes an excellent very rich moisturiser. It's a too rich for the face, but perfect for dry legs.

Other waxes such as olive, carnauba and jojoba waxes don't function as emulsifying ingredients. You can still use them in your skincare recipes, but only for their hardening and moisturising abilities.

ANTIOXIDANTS

Don't be confused into thinking that an antioxidant is a preservative. While antioxidants are known for keeping products fresher and extending their shelf life, they don't do this by preventing the growth of bacteria, yeast, fungus and mould. They aren't broad-spectrum preservatives, won't prevent the growth of bacteria and should not be confused with preservatives.

However, antioxidants do play two roles in your skincare products. One is to provide some protection against sun and environmental damage to the skin by neutralising free radicals, and the other is to help keep base oils from deteriorating and becoming rancid, therefore allowing the oils – and your skincare products – to stay fresher for longer.

Free radicals

Free radicals are caused by overexposure to sunlight, lack of sleep, pollution, stress, etc. Under normal conditions your body would work hard to replace these damaged cells with healthy new ones, but if free radicals aren't controlled or eliminated, the cells aren't repaired, resulting in dull, dry, wrinkled and uneven skin tone. Antioxidants help to get rid of free radicals before they do too much damage. This is why they are absolutely vital in anti-aging skincare products, as they are proven to help reduce the signs of aging.

Antioxidants also help reduce the rate of oxidation in oils. Oxidation is a chemical process that occurs when oils are exposed to air. As soon as a bottle of oil has been opened, it is exposed to the air and the gradual process of oxidation is kicked off. Antioxidants will extend the shelf life of your oils, especially 'fragile' ones such as flaxseed, hemp, rosehip and evening primrose oils.

Antioxidant ingredients

Many of the base oils, herbs, essential oils and other ingredients mentioned in this book have antioxidant qualities, some more than others.

Vitamin E

Vitamin E, also known as tocopherol, is a powerful antioxidant used in many skincare products, It not only helps the skin but it prevents the product itself from going rancid. Vitamin E can be added directly to your base oils to prevent them from becoming rancid in their bottles, or you can add it to your cosmetic products that contain these shorter shelf-life oils.

The ratio to use when adding vitamin E as an antioxidant to oils is about 1.5–2% This means that for every 1kg of base oil, you need to add 10g vitamin E.

Don't forget to label the bottle to remind yourself that it now contains vitamin E as well as the base oil.

Vitamin E is the perfect ingredient to add to rosehip oil because rosehip oil has a short shelf life and is known for its tendency to spoil fairly rapidly after opening. Adding 1g vitamin E oil to a 100ml bottle of rosehip oil will extend the shelf life of the oil to one to two years.

Rosemary oil extract

Rosemary oil extract is a powerful antioxidant. It also helps minimise the oxidation of some vitamins and amino acids. Because rosemary oil extract has a distinct smell of its own, you will introduce this aroma to your products if using it.

Green tea

Green tea has high levels of antioxidants and can be added to skincare products via a herbal infusion or an extract.

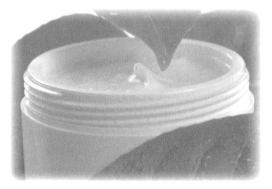

USING PRESERVATIVES

A preservative is an ingredient that stops the growth of bacteria and other micro-organisms. Preservatives are an important ingredient in cosmetic skincare preparations because the addition of a preservative allows the product to have an extended shelf life of up to two years or so.

As much as water is a vital ingredient in keeping us healthy and hydrated, in cosmetics water is, sadly, a breeding ground for bacteria. Therefore any cosmetic product containing water has a limited shelf life unless it has a reliable preservative system in place.

However, if you're creating small amounts of personal cosmetics that are to be used as soon as they are made, not using a preservative is an option. Commercially manufactured skincare products, by contrast, can be three months old or more before they even leave the warehouse, let alone land on a shop shelf or in your bathroom cabinet. For this reason, commercial skincare preparations contain preservatives to allow them to remain fresh, safe to use and non-toxic, from manufacture to the time the customer is finished using the product.

There has been some bad press in recent years about the safety of certain preservatives such as parabens and paraben derivatives. Typically this has led to a degree of wariness surrounding creams that contain this particular preservative (it should be noted that many of the parabens used are natural, however).

The most important characteristic of any cosmetic preparation is that it is safe to use. The fact of the matter is, products created without the use of preservatives have a limited shelf life, will go off and will start growing potentially dangerous organisms after time. To reduce, or even eliminate, the growth and volume of microorganisms, you need a preservative: enough to control microbial growth, yet not too much so as to cause allergies, dermatitis or any side effects.

What makes a good preservative?

A good preservative is one that can overcome the broad spectrum of microbes while ensuring that it doesn't harm the skin or have an adverse impact on any of the other ingredients a product contains.

A broad-spectrum preservative ensures that it prevents the growth of all kinds of bacteria, yeast, mould and fungus. A good preservative will be broad-spectrum and ensure that the growth of these unwanted micro-organisms is suppressed for the duration of a product's shelf life. A good preservative will also be safe for use on the skin, function properly within a wide pH range, work with other ingredients in the product that contains it and not cause any unnecessary smell or change to the product.

Preventing bacterial growth

Natural, preservative-free skincare products won't stay fresh for as long as commercial ones. Making your products in small batches that are used within a short period of time helps avoid the need for preservatives. You can also adopt some sensible practices in order to minimise the introduction and growth of bacteria in your freshly made skincare products. These include the following.

- Be sure your hands, work surfaces and utensils are scrupulously clean when creating your products so you don't contaminate your batch.

- Store your products in a cool, dark place. Sunlight, heat and moisture all help to spoil your product over time.

- Use cool, boiled water, spring water or distilled water in your products.

- Ensure that your packaging is airtight. Some products may oxidise and go rancid when exposed to air.

- Avoid putting your fingers into your products. Bacteria on your fingers can be transferred in this way. Use a clean spatula, lolly stick or cotton bud instead.

- Store your creams in an airtight pump to eliminate the introduction of bacteria via the air or transference from fingers.

- Store your products in the fridge and ensure that they are labelled properly so that you know what they are and what their use-by dates are.

Natural preservatives

Are there any natural preservatives? The answer is yes and no. Most preservatives contain chemicals and these chemicals can be natural. So let me change the question to: 'Are there any natural preservatives that don't contain chemicals?'

Very few natural preservatives are sufficiently adequate to keep your products safe and bacteria-free for as long as an 'unnatural' one. Commercially produced skincare products are likely to be stored in warehouses, on shop shelves and in cupboards for up to three years (or more) and therefore need to be preserved as thoroughly as possible – which means chemical preservatives designed for longevity.

Natural preservatives may not be sufficient to get your products successfully through the 'challenge test': a requirement for products before they can be sold legally. However, some natural ingredients will be a threat to bacteria and therefore help your product have an extended, but still limited, shelf life. This is especially useful if you want to make personal skincare products in slightly larger batches.

Natural and easily obtainable ingredients that may help to keep your products fresher longer are essential oils that contain antibacterial properties, such as tea tree, rosemary and thyme, neem oil, vitamin E, vitamin C, grapefruit seed extract, rosemary extract, honey, sugar, lemon and salt. Essential oils are natural substances that can have excellent preservative properties, but they have yet to be used extensively to preserve cosmetic products. Some are powerful antiseptics that kill harmful bacteria without harming the human body. For example, the addition of a single drop of sweet orange essential oil to 50g of an emulsified water and oil product will probably keep bacteria at bay, providing you use good hygiene when storing and handling the product.

Grapefruit seed extract

Grapefruit seed extract is a natural antibiotic, antiseptic, disinfectant and preservative. It is used to promote healing. Grapefruit seed extract, according to published sources, is effective against more than 800 bacterial and viral organisms, 100 strains of fungi, and a large number of single- and multi-celled parasites.

While it appears to make an excellent and natural preservative, many skin types find it harsh and a skin irritant. My suggestion to you is to make up a small batch of your product using grapefruit seed extract as its preservative and patch test it in the crook of your elbow or behind your ear to make sure you find it suitable.

Which preservative to use?

Every cosmetic product that needs a preservative has different requirements. Several factors determine which preservative is best for a particular product.

- *Type of product* Leave-on creams need different levels of preservative than shampoos.

- *Use of product* An eye cream may require a different level and style of preservative than a lipstick.

- *Shelf life* The longer you want a product to last, the more preservative you need to use. Typically, if you have no preservative, a water-content product will last a few days to a few short weeks.

By adding a preservative such as grapefruit seed extract at 1%, you extend the shelf life from a few weeks to a few months. With the use of a recognised, suitable preservative such as Optiphen included at 1%, you extend your product's shelf life to one year.

Many brand-name preservatives are available from cosmetic ingredient suppliers, and all do pretty much the same job: they keep your product safe by preventing the growth of bacteria, mould, fungus and yeast. Don't be afraid to use a preservative! They are safe and effective if used properly. But regardless of whether you use one or not, keep product containers, your work surfaces, equipment, utensils and hands clean to help your products remain safe.

Phenoxyethanol

Phenoxyethanol is an extremely safe, tested preservative. However, in order to be totally effective as a preservative, phenoxyethanol needs to be used with another tested ingredient such as methylisothiazolinone, chlorphenesin or caprylyl glycol.

Microkill COS & Optiphen

Two branded products, Microkill COS and Optiphen, are a blend of phenoxyethanol and caprylyl glycol. Microkill COS also has chlorphenesin included. When purchasing these preservatives, your supplier should advise what quantities you should consider using them in. He should also be able to give you advice as to when to include the preservative during the product-making session, and if there are any products for which the preservative isn't suitable. In general, usage rates are:

- 0.5–1% – will give your skincare product a 1-year shelf life

- 1–1.5% – will give your skincare product a 2–3 year shelf life

- 1.5% – is the maximum usage level.

Potassium sorbate

Potassium sorbate is a mild preservative used to suppress mould and yeast growth and is often found in food products and wine. It is made by reacting sorbic acid with potassium hydroxide and can be effective in skincare products with a typical pH of 5.5 or under. The usual amount added for adequate preservation is between 0.2 and 0.3%.

Non-water products

Cosmetic products that do not contain water are unlikely to require the addition of a preservative because no water is present to encourage bacteria growth. Products such as oil-based salves, facial oils, oil cleansers and serums will have a natural shelf life of a year or more, providing they are used and stored properly.

When a product has 'gone off'

The first thing you're likely to notice is furry spots of greyish-green mould growing on the product's surface. Other indications may be an 'off' or rancid smell or that the product stings a bit and has become too acid on your skin. This is due to a change in pH, the product's acidity level.

A product may discolour or turn cloudy when it was previously clear. It may also become thinner and liquid when it used to be a thick cream. Throw away a product if you believe it has gone off.

LIZ EARLE
CLEANSE & POLISH™
HOT CLOTH CLEANSER

NATURALLY ACTIVE INGREDIENTS

ROSEMARY, CHAMOMILE,
COCOA BUTTER AND
EUCALYPTUS ESSENTIAL OIL

CLARINS
PARIS

Capital
Jour

CLARINS
PARIS

Baume
té Éc

Boots

time delay

ANTI-AGEING

Wrinkle Reduce

NIGHT CREAM

CHAPTER 10

Commercial Skincare Products

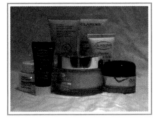

Many of the big brand-name skincare products contain similar ingredients to those you've been reading about in this book. Many also include other natural or less-than-natural ingredients that you have yet to experiment with in your quest to make skincare products.

Many commercially available skincare products include synthetic non-active ingredients, each designed to enhance the look, feel, smell and behaviour of the product itself, or simply just to add bulk. This not necessarily a bad thing, since each formulation has to be approved by a toxicologist and tested thoroughly to ensure that the combination of ingredients included is safe to go on the skin.

INCI names

The ingredients used in each product should be clearly identified in the ingredients list that will form part of the package labelling. If you read through such a list however, you may not initially recognise many ingredients. This is because the ingredients are listed under their INCI name, or International Nomenclature of Cosmetics Ingredients, which is a universally recognised system used on cosmetic product labels regardless of the language of the country where they are manufactured or sold.

In order to help you recognise the ingredients used in this book, I have included a list of some of them using both their common names and INCI names. When reading a label, remember that the ingredient that has been included in the greatest quantity will appear at the top, working down towards the ingredient used in the least amount.

If you're unsure of the translation of any of INCI names on labels, use Google as your first point of reference. Enter the INCI name into Google and with a bit of luck, the search results will tell you what the ingredient is in its more common form.

Common name	INCI name	Common name	INCI name
Almond (Sweet) Oil	Prunus amygdalus dulcis	Grapeseed Oil	Vitis vinifera
Apricot Kernel Oil	Prunus armeniaca	Hazelnut Oil	Corylus avellana
Argan Oil	Argania spinosa	Hemp seed Oil	Cannabis sativa
Avocado Oil	Persea gratissima	Honey	Mel
Bamboo Powder	Bambusa arundinaceae	Jojoba Oil	Simmondsia chinensis
Beeswax	Cera alba (white wax)	Jojoba Wax	Simmondsia chinensis
	Cera flavia (yellow wax)	Juniper Berry	Juniperus communis
Bergamot	Citrus aurantium bergamia	Kukui Nut Oil	Aleurites moluccana
Blackcurrant Seed Oil	Ribes nigrum	Lavender	Lavandula angustifolia
Carrot Seed	Daucus carota sativa	Lemon	Citrus limonum
Castor Oil	Ricinus communis	Lemon Grass	Cymbopogon schoenanthus
Cedarwood	Cedrus atlantica	Lime	Citrus aurantifolia
Chamomile	Anthemis nobilis	Macadamia Nut Oil	Macadamia ternifolia
Clary Sage	Salvia sclarea	Mango Butter	Mangifera indica
Clay	Kaolin or Bentonite	Melon Seed Oil	Citrillus lanatus
Cocoa Butter	Theobroma Cacao	Myrrh	Commiphora myrrha
Coconut Oil	Cocos nucifera (solid)	Neroli	Citrus aurantium
	Caprylic/Capric	Olive Oil	Olea europea
	triglyceride (liquid)	Orange (Sweet)	Citrus aurantium dulcis
Dead Sea Mud	Maris limus	Patchouli	Pogostemon cablin
Emulsifying Wax NF	Cetearyl alcohol (and)	Peach Kernel Oil	Prunus persica
	Polysorbate 60	Petitgrain	Citrus aurantium amara
Eucalyptus	Eucalyptus globulus	Rapeseed Oil	Brassica campestris
Evening Primrose Oil	Oenothera biennis	Rice bran Oil	Oryza sativa
Flaxseed Oil	Linum usitatissimum	Rose	Rosa damascena
Frankincense	Boswellia carteri	Rosehip Oil	Rosa canina
Geranium	Pelargonium graveolens	Rosemary	Rosmarinus officinalis
Grapefruit	Citrus grandis	Rosewood	Aniba rosaeodora

Common name	INCI name	Common name	INCI name
Sandalwood	Santalum album	Vitamin E Oil	Tocopherol
Safflower Oil	Carthamus tinctorius	Walnut Oil	Juglans regia
Shea Butter	Butyrospermum parkii	Water	Aqua
Sunflower Oil	Helianthus annuus	Wheatgerm Oil	Triticum vulgare
Tea Tree	Melaleuca alternifolia	Ylang-ylang	Cananga odorata

Allergens

You may see a few other ingredients occurring regularly on labels of products that contain essential oils. These are naturally occurring allergens. Those that need to be listed are: benzyl alcohol, benzyl salicylate, cinnamyl alcohol, cinnamal, citral, coumarin, eugenol, geraniol, isoeugenol, anise alcohol, benzyl benzoate, benzyl cinnamate, citronellol, farnesol, limonene and linalool.

While these may sound a little unfriendly, they are simply the individual components of many of the essential oils that help to shape their character, give them their wonderful aroma and enable them to have health-giving properties that our skin can take advantage of.

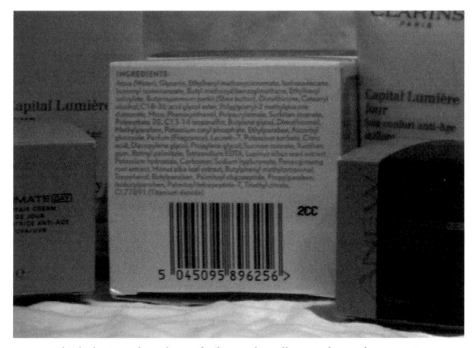

Check the ingredient list to find out what allergens the product contains

Resources

All of the ingredients, packaging and equipment needed to make the skincare products outlined in this book can be obtained online. Do keep an eye out for the ingredients in your local supermarket, too, as many of the oils and some of the floral waters are also used in cooking.

Training courses, kits, ingredients and packaging
Plush Folly
www.plushfolly.com
Tel: 07851 429 957

Ingredients and packaging
Gracefruit
www.gracefruit.com
Tel: 01324 841 353

The Soap Kitchen
www.thesoapkitchen.co.uk
Tel: 01805 622944

NHR Organic Oils
www.nhrorganicoils.com
Tel: 0845 310 8066

Exotic butters and oils
Shea Butter Cottage
www.sheabuttercottage.co.uk
Tel: 0208 144 4609

Of A Simple Nature
www.ofasimplenature.co.uk
Tel: 01372 726 523

Essential oils
Freshskin
www.freshskin.co.uk
Tel: 07846 174 876

ID Aromatics
www.idaromatics.co.uk
Tel: 0113 242 4983

Specialist herbs, gums and resins
Baldwins
www.baldwins.co.uk
Tel: 020 7703 5550

Organic Herb Trading
www.organicherbtrading.com
Tel: 01823 401 205

Grow-your-own fresh herbs
Jekka's Herb Farm
www.jekkasherbfarm.com
Tel: 01454 418 878

Bottles and packaging
Dormex
www.dormex.co.uk
Tel: 01928 703 160

Coloured bottles
www.colouredbottles.co.uk
Tel: 01634 862 839

Index

Also by Sally Hornsey

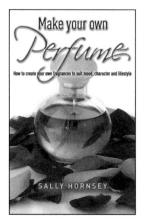

Make Your Own Perfume
How to create your own fragrences to suit mood, character and lifestyle

Wearing perfume is often limited by the cost of designer brands. Blending your own fragrances takes perfume-wearing to another level. You can design your own perfume to suit your mood, your character and your lifestyle – and, of course, your budget!

Make Your Own Perfume guides you through individual aromas, showing you how to design and structure perfume for yourself and for others. It includes blending tips to help you create your own range of gorgeous signature scents and fragrances that you can wear as often as you like.

In this book you will discover how to:

- Identify the fragrance families and choose which ones are better suited to different occasions
- Classify both natural and synthetic oils into 'note' categories to enable you to balance your perfume
- Make tinctures and infusions to use in your perfumes
- Dilute your perfume blend to become a body spray, eau de toilette, eau de parfum, pure perfume, or aftershave
- Package your perfume – and choose appropriate names for it
- Create perfume blends for potpourri, diffusers and other room-scenting products

Sally Hornsey runs Plush Folly, a private cosmetic training company specialising in a range of cosmetic-making workshops, kits, and home study courses. Sally's interest in perfume began when she managed the perfume counter for a well-known department store. Since then, her nose has taken her on a perfume adventure, and she enjoys having beautiful aromas and fragrances woven into her life. Sally has blended perfumes with celebrities on the radio and on television, and worked with members of the England Rugby team to create an April Fool's spoof aftershave that actually smelled good (even though it contained essence of sweaty sock!).

ISBN 978-1-905862-69-6